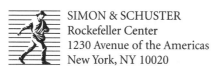

SIMON & SCHUSTER
Rockefeller Center
1230 Avenue of the Americas
New York, NY 10020

SIMON & SCHUSTER and colophon are registered trademarks of Simon & Schuster, Inc.

MAKE THE CONNECTION and GET WITH THE PROGRAM are registered trademarks of Harpo, Inc.

For information about special discounts for bulk purchases,
please contact Simon & Schuster Special Sales at
1-800-456-6798 or business@simonandschuster.com

This publication contains the opinions and ideas of the author. It is intended to provide helpful and informative material on the subjects addressed in the publication. It is sold with the understanding that the author and publisher are not engaged in rendering medical, health, psychological, or any other kind of personal professional services in the book. If the reader requires personal medical, health or other assistance or advice, a competent professional should be consulted.

The author and publisher specifically disclaim all responsibility for any liability, loss, or risk, personal or otherwise, that is incurred as a consequence, directly or indirectly, of the use and application of any of the contents of this book.

Designed by Nancy Singer Olaguera

Manufactured in the United States of America

10   9   8   7   6   5

Library of Congress Cataloging-in-Publication Data

Greene, Bob.
  Bob Greene's total body makeover / Bob Greene.
    p. cm.
  Includes index.
  1. Health. 2. Physical fitness. 3. Nutrition. 4. Weight loss. I. Title: Total body makeover. II. Title.

RA776.G7895 2005
613.7—dc22

                                              2004056601

ISBN 0-7432-5405-8

With special thanks to Daryn Eller and Michael Pool.

CONTENTS

BOB GREENE'S

TOTAL BODY
MAKEOVER

INTRODUCTION

Twelve weeks to total transformation. If you're familiar with *Get With the Program!, Make the Connection,* and Basic Training, a program on my Web site www.getwiththeprogram.org, you know that I've always said that it takes time and patience to lose weight. Now here I am with a three-month program. Have I gone off the deep end?

Not at all, and I think you'll agree when I explain the thinking behind Total Body Makeover.

Anytime I work with someone, be it on a one-to-one basis or through my books, my goal is to help that person attain physical health and emotional well-being. The 12-week Total Body Makeover is simply an accelerated program. It's a bit like boot camp: intense and meant to accomplish a lot in a short amount of time while giving you quicker and more dramatic results. One (and the most important) of those results is obtaining a new, elevated, and healthier metabolism. Through a combination of vigorous exercise and five simple eating rules—no strict or formal "dieting"—you will be burning far more calories each day when you reach the end of the 12 weeks.

This program offers something for everyone. Whether you're a beginning exerciser, already have a regular workout routine going, or are at an advanced level of fitness, you can personalize the Total Body Makeover plan to suit you. And no matter whether you have a substantial amount of weight to lose, a little to lose, or are just trying to get into the best shape of your life, you will see substantial changes in your body at the end of 12 weeks. Some of you will have reached your ultimate goal by then; some of you will have made a great start and will still have a way to go. But all of you, if you stay committed, will look and feel significantly different. Some of you will even have changed your lives in ways that were totally unexpected. Most important, you will be on the road to a lifetime of healthy living.

I can't stress enough how critical it is to have the proper mind-set before you begin this program. This means you have to think like an athlete. (You don't have to *be* an athlete, just think like one for now.) Athletes train intensely for an event, but once the event is over, they scale back and continue to stay active at a less rigid pace. That's essentially what you're going to be doing. You're going to ramp it up for 12 weeks, then pull back a bit but continue to be active and eat healthfully so that you don't lose the fitness, weight loss, and health strides you've made. Your goal should not be to follow this program for 12 weeks, celebrate the results, then abandon all the changes you made and return to what you were doing before. Granted, the 12 weeks are tough; I want to be honest about that. But I also want you to bear in mind that if you keep your goal in your line of sight, it will help you power through the days when staying on the program seems particularly difficult.

Here's what else I think will help you succeed on this program: the success of others. The pages of this book are peppered with stories of real-life people who have made over their bodies—indeed, their very lives—through their dedication and commitment. As you read these motivating tales, I hope they'll both inspire you and allow you to see your own struggles—and your own possibilities!—in the experiences of others.

To listen to the news these days is to hear some pretty dismal reports about Americans' ability (or rather, inability) to adopt healthy habits. Obesity rates are rising, large numbers of both kids and adults aren't exercising, many people find it hard to stick to a nutritious diet. And even when people do make an effort to slim down, they often give up after a while. According to some estimates, as many as 95 percent of people who lose weight gain it back. That's particularly scary when you consider that the latest figures indicate that obesity is fast on its way to replacing smoking as the number one cause of preventable death.

But there *are* people who are beating the odds and losing weight—

permanently. I know because I've met them. In my travels around the country, I've talked to many, many people who have committed themselves to change, with striking results. And they're not just slimming down for a few months, then ballooning back up again. They're dropping pounds and keeping them off over the long haul. That's the real challenge, and these inspiring individuals are meeting it.

As I see it, we all have a choice. We can dwell on the sad state of affairs and moan about how it must be impossible to be fit and healthy. Or we can take a look at those people who are successful and ask, What are they doing right? How did they overcome the obstacles that have tripped up so many others? We have so much to learn from these folks.

Certainly, in the grand scheme of things, the number of people who are able to lose weight and change their lives for good isn't staggering—it's really just a blip on the demographic chart that highlights the nation's expanding waistline. Nonetheless, each of the individuals you'll meet in this book proves that it's truly possible to effect significant change. And within each of their stories are some very important clues to how it's done. No two tales, as it turns out, are exactly alike, but every one of them shows that resolve can pay off.

Twelve Weeks to a New Body

Though the 12-week Total Body Makeover program is challenging on many levels, it doesn't include a formal diet. That may both surprise you and alarm you if that's the way you've tried to lose or control your weight in the past. But one of the things that sets my philosophy apart is that I firmly believe in getting an exercise program going and adopting a few simple eating rules: get a grip on your emotional eating, eat breakfast, have an eating cutoff time, drink plenty of water, and abstain from or limit your intake of alcohol—before you even begin to think about "officially" dieting. If you don't meet your goals, you may feel that you need to go on a structured eating plan when the 12 weeks are up. With this in mind I have devoted a lot of space in chapter 5 to helping you make sense of the most popular diets. However, right now it's in your best interest not to drastically cut calories before you have had a chance, through exercise, to ensure that your metabolism is running on high. And this may be particularly true if your metabolism, owing to the effects of going on diet after diet through the years, is as slow as molasses. Everybody can benefit from a metabolic charge-up before they start dieting, but chronic dieters *especially* need exercise to increase their calorie-burning rate.

Greatly restricting your food intake does the opposite of boosting your metabolism: it slows it down. The body is very sensitive to calorie input. Cutting way back on the amount of calories you consume triggers a survival mechanism, which developed when food was a lot scarcer than it is now and which causes your metabolism to switch into lower gear so that you don't expend energy too quickly. In fact, one of the *worst* things you can do is to restrict your calorie intake drastically without exercising at all. Because exercise can help moderate the body's survival tactic a bit, dieting at the same time you're exercising regularly is a little better, but, it's still not optimal. Best of all—and this is the approach built into this program—is to avoid formal dieting altogether, concentrate on exercise, and let the five simple eating rules in chapter 4 guide your approach to eating. While the rules may help you reduce your calorie intake a bit, you won't eat so little that your fat-defending survival mechanism kicks in.

Here's another important consideration: When you're in the throes of an intensive exercise program, you need to make sure you're getting enough calories to fuel your workouts. Go on a very-low-calorie diet, and you may feel too weak to work out!

When I tell my clients that they won't be dieting, some of them balk at first, but I ask them to be patient in order to see how well they do with just exercise and the eating and drinking guidelines first. The vast majority of them end up reaching their goals without ever having to go on a formal diet. Generally what happens is that after a certain point—it could be week two, it could be week four, it could be even after the 12 weeks are over—they reach a point I call the "free fall," when their metabolism revs up and the weight starts consistently melting off. Some people, though, even if they do eventually go into the free fall, don't lose enough weight. A small percentage of people find that they ultimately do need a structured plan to help them reach their goal.

I'm asking the same thing of you that I ask of my clients: Follow the 12-week program, *then* decide whether you need to follow a formal eating plan. I do think that under the right circumstances, diets can be very helpful, which is why I go over ten of the most popular ones in chapter 5, "Making the Transition to Real Life." They can assist you in clarifying your dietary needs and learning to make better food choices. Some of them will introduce you to a whole new way of eating that you never knew would be satisfying.

But whether you end up going on a diet or not, I think it's important to keep in mind that exercise has some revitalizing benefits that dieting, and especially going on a very rigid diet, doesn't. Working out is a proactive approach to reshaping your body. It's something you *do*, something you add to your life, and something that you'll quite possibly find can even be pleasurable. On the flip side, cutting calories is about *not doing* something, and, to me at least, that seems a lot harder, not to mention a lot less fun. I also believe that exercising combined with sensible eating is a much more effective, healthier—and ultimately more life-changing— approach than trying to diet your way there.

I can think of no better example of this than the struggle Oprah went through many years ago. Some of you may remember that she went on a liquid diet in 1988 and, in four months, lowered her weight from 211 to 142. She even came out on her show pulling a wagonful of lard representing all the body fat that she had lost. But something didn't seem right back then, and something wasn't. If you look at pictures of Oprah at that time, she was thin, but she had a gaunt appearance, and she certainly didn't have the muscle tone and healthy glow that she has today—seventeen years later!

Oprah's new body was short-lived. A year later, she was up to 175; a year and a half later, she hit an all-time high of 237 pounds. Needless to say, she was devastated.

Several years and life lessons later, Oprah looks healthy, vibrant, and radiant. If you saw pictures of her around the time of her fiftieth birthday in April 2004, you might have noticed that she has a new energy and vibrance. This time, she totally made over her body with exercise and sensible eating. She doesn't count calories, and she certainly hasn't been on a formal diet in a long, long time.

Conscientious eating and dieting are not the same thing. Conscientious eating is a way of life that allows you to stay within healthy boundaries while still eating enough to give you energy to exercise and to feel satisfied. Dieting is typically something you do short term, usually yielding short-term results. Sometimes going on a formal eating plan (though not an extreme one like a liquid diet) can really help you organize your eating and develop positive eating habits. Just be mindful that diets are not the be-all and end-all.

Now let's talk about exercise, the heart and soul of this program. There are actually three different categories of exercises you'll be doing over the 12 weeks: functional exercise, strength training exercise, and aerobic exercise. It may sound like a lot, but the three types of exercises are woven together smoothly so that in the end the combination feels like a seamless workout. From my experience working with many different people, I can tell you that it's very doable.

The first type of activity, functional exercises, refers to moves that improve your core strength, flexibility, balance, and coordination. They are primarily stretches and exercises that strengthen the stabilizing muscle groups, such as your abdominals. Through these moves, you'll achieve what's called functional fitness, which will not only make the strengthening and aerobic portions of the program easier for you to perform but also improve your posture, make you move more gracefully, and help you avoid injury.

To build strength, you'll be doing weight-training exercises, mostly with dumbbells or weight machines. These exercises will also help you increase your muscular power and endurance and, most important, strengthen your joints so that you can participate in more vigorous exercise. Strength training will also help you avoid injury and keep your metabolism running in high gear by building muscle. Muscle burns considerably more calories than body fat, increasing your body's calorie-burning potential.

The type of aerobic exercise you will do during this program will be your choice (although I'll have some recommendations for you). Aerobic workouts, the kind that elevate your heart rate, help you burn calories while you're doing them, of course, but they also boost your metabolism for hours after you've hung up your gym shoes. These workouts will be a critical part of your regimen, both for their weight loss and their health benefits.

Preparing for This Program

For many people, the preparation they do before embarking on an exercise program is just as important as—maybe even *more* important than—the program itself. It's essential that you realize that the meter on this program doesn't start ticking the minute you finish this introduction. It will vastly increase your chances of success if you first do some emotional work to ensure that your heart and mind, not just your body, are ready to go. The first chapter in this book, "Building a Sound Emotional Foundation," is dedicated to helping you lay the groundwork for change. In my experience, very few people have transformed their bodies without doing four things: telling themselves the truth about why they haven't been able to lose weight or get fit in the past; taking responsibility for their behavior; making a commitment to do what it takes to change; and mustering their inner strength to make it all happen. If you want to succeed in making your body over—indeed, if you want to succeed at life—here are the keys to the castle.

What these four cornerstones—honesty, responsibility, commitment, and inner strength—do is provide a rock-solid emotional foundation that will hold you up when the going gets rough. And it will. Without these four cornerstones, trying to institute change is like building a house on an unstable foundation—at the first rumble of trouble, it's likely to tumble.

Changing your behavior isn't easy, but it's a lot easier if you have a very good sense of yourself as well as an unwavering dedication to your goal. People who succeed look themselves in the eye and are truthful about why they are where they are in their lives. They identify their weaknesses and their discomforting or painful personal issues, and they make the connection between them and their eating habits and inactivity. If they're overweight, they dig down deep to understand why. When they figure out what it is that needs to change, they make a promise to their harshest critic—themselves—to change it and muster the willpower to see it through.

I'm not discounting the fact that you may already have a strong emotional foundation. Many people are already clear about what they're doing wrong and staunchly committed to doing what it will take to fix it. If you haven't started a bunch of other programs only to fail again and again and you feel that you have the resolve and the willpower to do what it takes to succeed, you can give chapter 1 a pass—or, better yet, quickly read it to reinforce where you are.

If, on the other hand, you *have* experienced failure many times, you can't pass this chapter by. I wish it were the case that all you had to do to get the body you want is to get onto a treadmill or pick up some weights, but experience has shown me that it's almost impossible to lose weight (or, more precisely, to keep lost weight from returning) if you don't address why you are overweight in the first place, whether it's a deep-seated emotional matter, lack of support from those around you, simple bad habits, maybe even just laziness. Excess weight is always a symptom of something else. Identifying what that something else is and changing it is the key to long-term success. If you address only the symptom, you'll never permanently solve the problem.

The time you spend preparing your mind to tackle the big job of changing your body will be time well spent. I've quite often met people who have lost more than 150 pounds, totally transforming the way they look and, most important, the way they feel about themselves. I have talked to men and women who, though they needed to lose only a small amount of weight, used exercise to help them achieve a total health overhaul. I've also met people who, by most standards, already lived a healthy life but who wanted to become—and did become—superfit. What these people all had in common was that they achieved their goals when—and only when—they were completely ready. Many of them had tried and failed many times before, but at some point they pulled themselves up by their bootstraps, turned a searching eye on their lives, and came away with the insight, willpower, and commitment they needed to succeed. It's not as though once they made the decision, they never experienced a temptation to return to their old ways—that, to be honest, never goes away. But they became better at managing their lives and, consequently, better at fending off the pull of anything that would get in the way of their success.

It's not enough to want to transform your body; everybody wants to do that. You have to want to do the hard work that is required to lose weight. Tough decisions will be required of you, and you have to be ready, even eager, to make them. No one succeeds without giving up something, be it leisure time or favorite foods. You may find that you even have to revaluate and change some of the relationships you're in.

But let me tell you that the sacrifices you make in the process of transforming yourself will change your life drastically and, usually, in the best way possible. That, in fact, should be your biggest motivator next to wanting to improve your health. The way you feel about yourself (the way you feel, period), your relationships with others, your whole approach to the world can be different and far more positive. I haven't yet met anyone who successfully made their body over without finding that their lives changed in ways—wonderful ways—that they had never imagined.

The prospect of shaking up your world may not sound all that interesting when you're really just thinking about how to lose 5 or 50 or even 150 pounds. That's okay; let the weight loss be your focus, but keep the prospect of life changes in the back of your mind, because ultimately, it's probably going to happen, and if you're like any of the successful people you'll be reading about in this book, you'll be thrilled that it did.

What Else Is in Store?

As part of your preparation for the 12-week program, I'd like you to put your intentions into writing by signing a contract with yourself. If you're familiar with some of my other books or if you've seen my work with people on *The Oprah Winfrey Show,* you'll know that I often ask people to sign contracts with *themselves.* Why? For the simple reason that it can really make a difference in the way you approach change. Putting something into writing gives what's being promised greater weight, especially when the person you are making the promise to is you. Signing a contract also creates something tangible that you can drag out and put on the table as a constant reminder that you are committed to making your body over. You probably wouldn't break a contract you had with someone else; my hope is that you'll also be true to the contract you make with yourself.

In January 2003, *O, The Oprah Magazine* published a contract I designed (similar to the one in this book) that challenged readers to commit themselves to regular exercise, healthful food choices, and nutritional rather than emotional eating. The idea was to take people a step beyond the usual "Yeah, I'm going to do something about my health." Thousands of women (and men) sent in contracts, and while I can't claim to know how it worked for all of them, many followed up with letters telling us that signing the contract had been a turning point in their lives and that they'd gone on to keep the commitment. They proved that making a promise, in writing to yourself, can be a positive catalyst for change.

I also want to talk a bit about emotional eating. In a perfect world, everyone would eat just enough to fuel them through their day and provide them with a nice amount of sensory pleasure. As it is, many people eat for emotional reasons—boredom, stress, anxiety, depression, a void in their lives. If you're one of them, it's important to identify and acknowledge the emotional trigger points that send you running to the refrigerator or the cupboard. This, too, is about telling yourself the truth. What are your real feelings, and why are you trying to mask them with food? In chapter 3, you'll find some tools to help you answer these questions and avoid burying emotional issues under boxes of cookies and cartons of ice cream. For many people, simply eliminating emotional eating can be the difference between weighing 250 pounds and 125 pounds, no dieting involved.

If you do end up going on a diet, it's crucial to pick the right one. I don't believe in one-size-fits-all diets. People are different. Some need a lot of structure; some need a little structure or none at all. But one thing is true for everybody: in order for a diet to work, you have to stay on it, and in order for you to stay on it, it has to realistic and within your capabilities. It has to suit your tastes, your lifestyle, and your resources. Not your sister's, a friend's, or some movie star's, but yours. And since only you can know what type of eating plan will fit you to a T, I want you to be in charge of selecting your own diet—though I've done some legwork to help guide you toward one that will safely allow you to continue your body makeover process.

In chapter 5, "Making the Transition to Real Life," I'll take a look at popular eating plans: What do they really ask of you? What are their advantages and disadvantages? Who will they probably work best for? I also want to give you the option of developing your own plan. If you already know what type of eating plan works for you, and as long as your self-devised diet isn't drastic or unhealthy (an earlier book of mine, *The Get With the Program Guide to Good Eating*, can help you establish some parameters), go for it. What counts is that it be a plan you can stick with.

Keep in mind that the science of nutrition and weight loss is relatively young. We are always learning new things about the body and how it reacts to food and exercise, so the definitive ultimate diet is probably quite a few years away. That said, there are some fundamental truths about becoming healthier and slimmer. One of them is that not everybody has to follow the same exact diet plan in order to succeed at losing weight. In fact, different people respond differently to different diets, although nobody is exactly sure why. Some people, for instance, feel energetic and full of life while following a low-carbohydrate diet, while others feel as though they can barely muster the energy to get off the couch. Some people feel hungry all the time on a low-fat diet, while others feel perfectly satisfied. Some people drop a ton of weight when given an exact menu for every meal; others, oddly enough, end up gaining.

That said, bear in mind that the formula for weight loss is fairly simple: When the calories coming in (what you eat) are fewer than the calories going out (what you expend through exercise, basic body functions such as your heart beating and eyes blinking, and unstructured activity such as brushing your hair out of your eyes), you will lose weight. No matter what eating plan you end up choosing, that's the bottom line.

Tawni: The Amazing Woman on the Cover of This Book

If you need a muse to get you started on the road to total transformation, I recommend Tawni, the incredible woman I am posing with on the cover of this book. I'll let Tawni tell you her story in her own words, but let me preface it by saying that she is proof of that old saying "Where there's, a will there's a way."

A Lightbulb Goes On
Tawni's Story

Like a lot of people who struggle with their weight, I had been heavy most of my life, having had only a brief period of "normal" weight during high school. But the way I stayed thin back then was hardly normal: my mom sent me to a "fat farm," where I lost a bunch of weight, and then I kept it off by forcing myself to vomit after eating binges. During my senior year I kicked the purging habit, but the binging continued. Eventually I gained 50 pounds.

After high school and throughout my twenties, I turned to food for comfort. I was depressed and lonely, and food soothed me. But it was a vicious cycle. I'd feel depressed, eat, then feel depressed about eating. By the time I moved to San Francisco in 1994, I weighed almost 185 pounds, quite a bit for someone who is only five feet, three inches tall.

To make matters worse, while I was in the process of moving I was carjacked. Everything I owned except for the clothes on my back was taken, and I had to start over from scratch. Add to that the fact that I was in a new city where I knew no one, and the loneliness was nearly intolerable. Again I turned to food for solace. That first year in San Francisco, I gained more than 100 pounds, hitting 295.

Change eventually started to come, but it came slowly. I began to get my bearings. I bought clothes and furniture, and started to rebuild my life.

In 1996, I was on a business trip in Arizona. When I got back to my hotel room and flipped on the TV, *The Oprah Winfrey Show* was on. It wasn't the first time I'd watched: I'm a huge fan of Oprah's, and I had a habit of taping the show every day. On that particular afternoon, I stayed put and watched the show, which was about the launch of *Make the Connection*, a book that Oprah and Bob had written together.

I sat in that hotel room and couldn't believe what I was hearing. Oprah gets up at 5 A.M. to exercise? I bought the book and stayed up all night in my hotel room reading it. The book appealed to me because it wasn't a diet, it was a way of life. It was about working from the inside out, and it dawned on me that that was always the way I had known I was going to lose weight.

What happened in that hotel room is that I had an honest conversation with myself. I admitted to myself that if one of the most industrious women in America was making time to exercise, my own excuse was lame. After some soul-searching, I owned up to the idea that I didn't need a magic diet; I needed something that would help me address my emotional eating.

When I got back to San Francisco, I bought a treadmill, put it right in front of the TV in my tiny apartment, and started walking every evening after work while I watched a tape of Oprah's daily show. That was in September. By December I'd lost 20 pounds.

Then, on December 4, I got up early to do my walking routine outside for the very first time. (I'd never stopped thinking about Oprah getting up at five and wondering if I too could become a morning person.) Luck wasn't with me: I was hit by a car and spent the next six months in a wheelchair while going through rehab.

It might have been a serious setback, but this time, unlike after the carjacking incident, I decided to come out better, not bitter. I was feeling good about the 20 pounds I'd lost and didn't want another 100-pound gain. I'd been honest with myself about my past behavior and was successfully using it to predict—and prevent—my future behavior. (Because, for instance, I knew I tended to overeat when stressed, when heading into a stressful situation I'd bring baby carrots or celery to munch on so I wouldn't make a beeline for the vending machines.)

In addition, I had founded a support group for people struggling with their weight, and I was the leader. I needed to set a good example; I didn't want to let the group down. Something else was also different this time around. While in the beginning, losing the weight had taken a lot of willpower, now the things that had allowed me to succeed—lots of exercise and retooling my diet—had become habit. I was in the habit of healthy living.

My group helped me as much as I helped them. Through the power of the group and my conviction that I wouldn't be a victim this time around, I didn't gain an ounce during the six months after the accident. As soon as I got out of the wheelchair, I picked up with my walking right where I'd left off. Three months later, I did my first 5K run.

By 1998, I had lost more than 100 pounds. I weighed 175 and was proud of it. I'd done it slowly and consistently by cleaning up my diet and exercising. Ironically, although I'd gone through years of therapy to combat depression and even tried antidepressants, exercise turned out to be the best drug for me—and all the side effects were positive ones.

This isn't the end of my story. I won my weight loss battle because I made a commitment to myself to not let anything stand in my way—and I held to it. Last year I even renewed my commitment and signed the "Contract with Myself." [The same contract you'll find on page 58.] My goal this time was to lose enough weight to run the Chicago Marathon in October in under five hours. Today, I have 30 marathons under my belt and weigh 140 pounds.

This process took me eight years. I had my setbacks and even some tragedies in between. But it has all been worth it because I have changed not just my body, but almost every aspect of my life. While I've always been an overachiever, before this transformation, my personal life was out of control. I always initiated contact with both men and women friends, and I'd jump through hoops to please them. Underneath there was a lot of envy and resentment in these relationships. Now I have healthier, more balanced relationships. Whereas I used to never take time for myself, now I make it a priority. I'm asked to do fifty million things a day, but now before I say yes I look at how it's going to affect the things that I have to get done for me. I'm no longer last on my list.

Another big change in my life has been a newfound ability to speak my mind. It used to be that if my husband's socks were on the floor, I'd get resentful and go eat a bowl of ice cream. I never made the connection that I was eating because I was upset. Now instead of eating I just say, "Would you pick up your socks?" I stand up for myself and say what I think. If I'm uncomfortable with something, I say so. If someone hurts my feelings, I tell them. I also now use exercise as an outlet for my feelings. I used to be an emotional eater; now I'm an emotional exerciser. I even keep an emergency pair of shoes in my car so that if I get stressed out I can pull over and walk instead of pulling into the closest drive-through. I used to nervously eat, now I nervously walk.

I've learned to set new boundaries and make decisions that

aren't always popular. Before I was married, my friends weren't too happy when I told them I couldn't go out to clubs because I had to be asleep by ten so I could get up early and exercise. But that's all part of it. I worked hard for every pound I lost, and I still do. Along the way I discovered that my real passion and joy in life is helping others find the same happiness I have. Through two Web sites that I run (www.nomoreexcuses.net and www.connectingconnectors.com), I have become part of a whole new community.

You might say that Tawni is a marathoner in more than one sense of the word. Just as she has run races, taking them step by step and staying the course, so has she improved her life by changing it bit by bit and hanging in there over the long haul. Like marathoning, making your body over is a test of endurance and one that you can succeed in only if you are willing to keep chugging along. The next 12 weeks will be a little bit of a sprint, but they're just part of the training for an ongoing process. When you cross the finish line, you'll be fitter than ever—and ready to stay on the path to a new life.

1

BUILDING A SOUND EMOTIONAL FOUNDATION

MOST PEOPLE POISED TO embark upon a 12-week body makeover program will begin by thinking about, and maybe even worrying about, how they're going to change their eating and exercise habits. But this program is different. It begins not with food or fitness, but with something that I think is equally, if not more, important: building a solid emotional foundation.

If you've tried lots of other weight loss programs before (and even if you haven't), putting diet and fitness concerns aside for a short while probably seems like a pretty crazy idea. In fact, it's the sanest thing you can do. If you want to transform your body, the first thing you need to do is transform your mind-set, your attitudes, your outlook, your way of seeing the world, and most critical of all, your way of seeing yourself.

The root of most people's weight problems, or any problems that relate to lack of motivation, is buried deep within. I have heard enough tales of stalled body makeover attempts to confidently say that virtually no one—no one—who hopes to lose weight and keep it off for good can succeed without first addressing her attitudes and the way it affects her behavior, then shoring up her level of motivation. You can cut calories and exercise all you want, but if you don't develop a strong emotional foundation first, everything you've built is likely to fall down like a house of cards. For long-term success, spend the time to make yourself emotionally healthy before you even think about adjusting your diet or joining a gym.

Building a new, healthier life for yourself is a lot like building a house: both require that you start by laying a foundation. Without a foundation to prop it up, a house cannot stand (at least for long). Likewise, without a strong emotional foundation, everything you achieve toward making your body over will not withstand the stress, strains, and temptations of daily life. The house, your body—each needs a solid base.

So how do you build that base? It starts with four cornerstones. You might call them the mental equivalent of bricks and mortar: honesty, responsibility, commitment, and inner strength. They're the seeds of success for accomplishment in weight loss and, in fact, all areas of life. The reason is very simple: these four cornerstones provide you with what you need to stay resolute in the face of everyday challenges to your resolve. They also help you weather the storms that typically derail months and even years of effort. If you think about it, when someone fails to reach a goal, it's usually because there's been a breakdown in one of these four areas. But if you've got them all in check and are standing on steady emotional ground, nothing—not relationship troubles, family crises, job stress, blows to your self-esteem, illness—is going to keep you from achieving long-term success.

I want you to know, though, that honesty, responsibility, commitment, and inner strength are more than just concepts. Each represents a goal in itself, one that can be reached only by doing some serious soul-searching and self-evaluation. Much is often made about how difficult it is to eat right and exercise, but taking an honest look at yourself and working to change or fortify some fundamental aspects of your personality is an even greater challenge. So by asking you to lay the four cornerstones of a strong emotional foundation, I am asking you to gear up for what might be a tough, challenging, and perhaps even uncomfortable endeavor. Getting there may or may not be fun— some people find that having those moments of self-revelation where everything comes together is quite wonderful, others don't.

But making the effort is entirely worth it.

Successful people who have made honesty, responsibility, commitment, and inner strength central to their very being have found that it changed them in ways they would never have imagined. That's because while, certainly, these are the keys to making your body over once and for all, they are also the keys to accomplishing *anything.*

As you go through the steps of conquering each cornerstone, you'll find you have the power to let go of the past and anything else that is stopping you from becoming the person you really want to be. I'm not going to kid you: the process can be rough. But make it through the emotional discomfort, and you'll find that you have emotional freedom and that the pleasure you can take in this empowering, life-changing experience will far outweigh the pain. If you're tired of feeling guilty about your actions and are disgusted with yourself for procrastinating, tired of feeling bad about the way you look, and fearful about the state of your health, this is the road you want to be on.

I want to qualify this a little bit before I go on. Just as there are exceptions to every rule, there are exceptions to the idea that most people need to do some soul-searching before they try to lose weight. Maybe you already have a good mind-set about eating and exercise, know yourself well, and take responsibility for your actions. Maybe you've just never had to be disciplined about eating and exercise before and simply need some help getting on to the right track. Perhaps committing to something isn't a problem for you as long as you have the right tools to work with. If you feel you don't need to spend the time working on your emotional foundation, then by all means move on to the next chapter. But it's not a bad idea to spend some time reading through the next sections just to reinforce the attitudes and actions that determine success (and failure).

So here's the deal: Take however long you need to be honest with yourself, assume responsibility for your actions, make a commitment to change your life, and use your inner strength to help you stick to your resolve. *Then* move on to the 12-week Total Body Makeover program and the task of achieving your goals. Believe me, years down the road, when you have transformed your body—and kept it that way— you won't regret taking this extra step in the least.

The First Cornerstone: Honesty

The process of change requires that you stop wearing blinders; you must be honest with yourself about who you are and why you do the things you do. It's funny how we can so often give an incisive psychological portrait of other people yet are frequently at pains to truly know ourselves. I'm asking you to be as insightful into your own psyche as you are into others'.

Lying to yourself is like having one big crack in your emotional foundation—you're in trouble before you even get started. I've met people who've made a career out of deluding themselves and as a consequence never really accomplished what they wanted to. By making excuses, blaming others, putting things off—and all the while telling themselves that they're not really doing the things that they are indeed doing—they have doomed themselves to failure.

I can't stress enough how essential being honest about your strengths, your weaknesses, and even your past failures will be to your success. Recently I met with a client who was reluctant to answer any of my questions about his life. I wasn't trying to be nosy or to be a trainer/therapist. I was just trying to get a read on some of the issues that might be affecting his weight. I respected his privacy and certainly understood that it's not easy to share the details of your life with someone you barely know. But I also told him that when it comes to what he tells *himself*, reticence is a different matter. He didn't have to tell me what was going on, but not being truthful with himself would be self-defeating.

An unwillingness to open up and to experience the discomfort that kind of honesty inevitably brings is a huge barrier to success. This process is about self-discovery, and those who go through it change not only the behaviors that previously kept them from dramatically altering their bodies but the behaviors that hampered their lives in other ways, too. Sometimes what you find out about yourself is embarrassing; sometimes it's painful; sometimes it's just depressing. But when you have that "Aha!" moment—"Oh, *that's* why I've been doing that!"—it can be very freeing. Imagine trying to fix a lamp that suddenly goes off without checking to see if the lightbulb is burned out. Your chances of getting the light back on aren't very high. Same thing here: if you've tried to lose weight again and again without determining what is fundamentally causing the problem, you're working in the dark. It's just not going to happen. Oh, you might lose the weight for a while, but before you know it, you're going to put it back on.

The point of doing some honest self-exploration is not to beat yourself up about your shortcomings. Rather, it's to learn something that you didn't know about yourself or, if you did know it on some level, to officially admit it to yourself. When you make these discoveries, it's important not to just gloss over them. Don't just tell yourself, "Yeah, I guess I stopped walking after work not because it was so late when I got home but because I really preferred to watch *Jeopardy!*" Pause and think more about it. Do you really like *Jeopardy!* that much, or are you using it as an excuse? Are you lazy? Are you embarrassed to be seen "fitness walking" around your neighborhood because you think it calls attention to your weight? Are you afraid that your significant other will be angry at you for taking the time for yourself? Do you simply have no energy (a problem that might be remedied by switching your workouts to the morning)? What is really going on? Your assignment is to find out. Replay decisions you've made, both good and bad, and analyze them. It's the only way you're going to break ingrained unhealthy behavior patterns.

Here's the story of how one client of mine did it. She asked herself some hard questions, and the answers helped her get onto the right track.

Who's Your Boss?
Abby's Story

A friend introduced me to Bob, and the two of us enlisted him to help us lose weight and get fit. I got off to a good start: six weeks into my program, my regular workouts and the changes I'd made in my diet were having a noticeable impact. But then things started to go wrong. I began missing some of my exercise sessions, and I had to confess to Bob that I wasn't making healthy meals as often as before. I didn't see this as my fault, though. My kids were rebelling against the new, healthier menu, and my husband was making snide remarks about there being nothing good to eat in the house. Even my mother-in-law made comments about me being away from home so much now that I was exercising.

When Bob asked me why I'd cut back on both my healthy meals and my workouts, I blamed it on all the other people in my life: my kids, my husband, my mother-in-law. He asked me if I really thought that it was their fault and not my own. I admitted that I have had a tendency to blame other people when things don't work. Bob then asked me to take a good hard look at the present situation and be truthful about it: If I were to keep foods in the house that would satisfy my kids and husband, did that mean I would have to eat them too? Couldn't I be frank with my mother-in-law about how much meeting my weight loss goals meant to me? I realized he was right and that I alone and no one else was in control of my situation.

Over the next few weeks, I made it a point to speak honestly with my family, and to my surprise they were very understanding once I made it clear what I was trying to do. It not only improved my relationship with everybody but also got them on my side. In just outside of a year, I met my weight loss goals.

Abby had been in denial for a long time, but by finally facing up to the truth about herself, she was able to recover her fitness gains and go on to achieve even more. What I'm suggesting, though, is that you *begin* by assessing where you're at so that you don't find yourself grappling with obstacles in mid-makeover. Abby recovered, but many people do not. They just end up back where they started, wondering why they can never get the body they want.

I'll tell you another reason why it's so important to be honest with yourself at the outset. I have had many clients who believed that they simply lacked the proper discipline to turn down their favorite foods, when in reality their dilemma was much more complex. Many people eat because something is missing from their lives, and they don't connect it to their bad eating habits. It may have been that they never took the time or wanted to expend the energy to explore their feelings. It may have even been that exploring their feelings was simply too discomforting or painful, so they buried those feelings away beneath platefuls of food.

Sometimes it's obvious when we lie to ourselves, but other times we are simply not self-aware. Either way, you can find the truth if you make an effort to investigate who you really are. Do you feel as though you are a victim of life's circumstances or do you feel that you have control of your life? What makes you happy? What makes you sad? Are your relationships with other people distressing or joyful? What is your family history like, and how has it influenced your behavior? Have you experienced something traumatic in the past, and, if so, what are the mechanisms you've developed to cope with it? Do you use food as an anesthetic to deal with emotional pain? If you do, why is food your drug of choice?

These are some of the hard questions you need to ask yourself. Many of the issues they touch on may be sore spots, but, the only way you're going to be able to move forward is to deal with the past, then find a way to put it behind you. Bury the truth, and you'll have cracks in your foundation before you even start building; grasp the reality of your own life, and you'll be on your way to changing your body and your health for the better.

Self-discovery, I should add, doesn't end when you reach a certain weight or size; it's an ongoing process. So even though the exercises that follow are aimed at helping you begin the task of learning the truth about yourself, you need to continue to honestly examine your attitudes and actions on an ongoing basis. Just as giving up on exercise or, say, returning to night eating can undo all the good that's been done, so can losing the self-awareness you develop at the outset of this program.

Finally, it's important to note that being honest with yourself also means telling the truth about your strengths, not just your weaknesses. Discovering and acknowledging your assets is part of the process because you're going to need to rely on those strengths to help you succeed. So as you go through the following exercises, be mindful of the positive features of your personality. We all have weaknesses, but we all have strengths, too.

Get to Know Yourself

People who are successful at weight loss have asked the hard questions and responded with straightforward answers. No rationalizations, no excuses. Instead of taking a cosmetic approach to the problem, they've gotten to the root of their behavior, making change possible. A weight problem or chronic unhappiness with your body isn't like a cut; you can't just put a bandage on it and hope that it will heal. While excess weight is evident on the exterior, it really stems from inside you, which means that you have to dig down deep to remedy the situation.

Recently I heard someone say that the hardest thing to do in baseball is to hit a pitch that's going 95 miles per hour. But people do it every day, he said, and the reason is that they know what's coming at them and can prepare for it. I think that's a perfect metaphor for this truth-telling process. Losing weight and keeping it off is one of the hardest things you can do, but the people who do it do so because they know what to expect. They know themselves, and they know how to prepare for their reactions in certain situations. Someone who knows herself will know that a family holiday dinner is going to make her revert back to her old ways of eating with childlike abandon, and she can prepare for it by bringing along healthful dishes that will help her control her portions. Someone who knows the truth about herself will know that she feels self-conscious in exercise classes—so she'll find an individual workout she likes or a trainer to work with instead. The more honest you are with yourself, the better you'll do on this program.

If you're at a loss as to where to begin, the following exercises will help. I've profiled eight of the most common types of behaviors that lead to failure and indicate a need for some soul-searching. If one or more of the behaviors sound all too familiar, it's a call for you to ask yourself some probing questions. I'll guide you by giving you some things to think about, but you need to rely on yourself for the answers. Be completely honest even if it hurts. Personally, I think that writing things down really aids in this kind of soul-searching, but whether you want to record the answers to the questions you ask yourself or just mull them over is up to you.

If you've read any of my other books, some of the questions might seem familiar: Do you procrastinate? Are you an immediate gratification junkie? Do you put the blame on other people and make excuses for why you don't eat right or exercise? I ask them again not because I lack imagination but because after talking to hundreds of people about their weight problems, I know that procrastination, the need for immediate gratification, blaming, excuse making, and all the other issues that this section deals with are exceptionally common. One or more of them is almost always at the core of an overweight person's predicament. And these issues cut across all lines—age, gender, race, profession, financial class. People from all walks of life deal with them.

This isn't to say that something other than the problems I identify here might be tripping you up. These exercises are limited in scope. Create other questions for yourself that are specific to your individual life. Think about things people have told you about yourself, both good and bad. Do they apply? Anything that allows you to discover more about yourself will help you with this endeavor. Believe me, the time you spend reflecting on what you think and feel will be time well spent.

I really want to drive that point home because many people feel that such exercises are a waste of time or that doing them is just not their style. Even a close friend told me that she had liked one of my earlier books but could never see herself doing the emotional exercises; she just wasn't the "type"—though *I* believed she was *exactly* the type of person who actually needed to do them the most. Interestingly, she recently began working with someone who gave her very similar exercises to try; she's been doing them and making progress. So even if you don't consider yourself the soul-searching type, give them a try. What have you got to lose?

Cutting Corners: Are you always looking for the easy way out?

In matters of traveling from, say, Albuquerque to Santa Fe, taking shortcuts may be a desirable, even wise plan of attack. In matters of changing your life, however, cutting corners is simply foolish. Much as I'd like to tell you that there's an easy way to lose weight and keep it off, there is no easy way.

Now, be honest—have you tried "miracle" schemes, diets, pills, or the like that promise to whittle your body down without any work on your part at all? Even if you haven't fallen for any of these gimmicks of the diet trade, ask yourself if you ever really work hard to achieve your goals. It doesn't even have to be weight loss–related. It could be anything, from something at work to something in your home life. Are you always looking to accomplish something by doing as little effort as possible? How many times have you taken shortcuts or done far less than your best when trying to achieve something? How did it work out? Were you satisfied with the results? Would you say you were successful? Be honest about why you took the easy route. Has it been a lifelong habit, or did something happen to change the way you approach a challenge? Ask yourself, too, why you cut corners. Out of laziness? Impatience? Fear of failing if you take a more challenging path?

To get anywhere in life, you have to be dedicated and hardworking. Cutting corners, on the other hand, is the sure road to failure. If you hope to accomplish anything worthwhile, you've got to do the work. And I don't just mean that you have to work at weight loss (though of course you do). Putting forth a valiant effort is the prime ingredient for success in everything, from maintaining a loving relationship and raising a family to advancing in a career. The hard workers succeed; the corner cutters typically do not.

So why aren't you working hard? If laziness is your problem, you need to pick yourself up and get going. Realize, too, that energy begets energy. You know the old saying "If you want something done, give it to a busy person"? The more you do, the more you *can* do, and I believe the same holds true when it comes to putting effort into reaching a goal. Once you get going, working hard will be easier for you. You'll get into it, and the lazy person in your past will seem like a stranger.

If impatience is your problem, consider that most accomplishments achieved overnight tend to fall apart just as rapidly. Patience, as they say, is a virtue, and while taking shortcuts may get you some rapid results, they're not results that will be likely to stick around. (See page 30 for more on the perils of immediate gratification.)

Some people cut corners for an entirely different reason: they feel that they're just not capable of doing the work. If that's true in your case, you've got to work on building your confidence. Believe in yourself! The work ahead may be hard, but you'll be taking it one step at a time, which will make it easier. Think of Tawni, whom you met in the introduction and who went from being bedridden to running marathons. She didn't jump out of bed and head for the finish line. She went step by step, building on each small success. That's what you're going to do, too.

Making Excuses: Do you always have a "reason" for not making good on your commitments?

Excuse makers are people who always, always find a reason for not doing what they've committed to do, whether that commitment was to themselves or to others. Excuse makers are never at a loss for a creative reason for their actions, but when you examine the justification it almost always breaks down.

Excuses are big obstacles in the road to change, though you may not even be aware that you're making them. Instead, you may just view them as "reasons." When you're late for an appointment or you break a promise to do somebody a favor, do you say, "I was late for lunch because of the traffic" when the real reason is "I was late for lunch because even though I know there is always traffic at this hour, I was talking on the phone and didn't leave early enough" and the bottom line was "I was late for lunch because I put my desire to continue a conversation before someone else's desire not to sit alone waiting at a table for a half hour"?

If you're capable of making excuses like that, you are probably also capable of making excuses for not exercising and eating right. How many times have you lied to yourself about why you didn't make it to the gym or why you ended up ordering a pizza for dinner? Do you tell yourself things like "Well, my ankle was kind of hurting" and "That's what the kids wanted for dinner" instead of admitting "I just didn't feel like working out" and "That's what *I* wanted for dinner"?

I think you know deep down when you're kidding yourself. Now's the time to own up to it and to investigate the real reasons behind your behaviors.

Excuses are a sure sign that you're not ready to do the hard work of change that lies in front of you. On the other hand, if you're willing to call yourself on your excuses and see them for what they are—diversionary tactics you're using to keep yourself from feeling awful about making bad choices or ways to defend your current way of life—then there's hope. You need to realize that making excuses affects not just you but others in your life. Sometimes excuses can be legitimate, but mostly they're just dishonest. If you're always giving yourself a pass (and asking other people to do the same), you're never going to get anywhere. So acknowledge your excuses past and present and resolve to remove them from your vocabulary.

People who succeed at weight loss give up on making excuses. They don't let themselves off the hook. They're not always perfect, but when they aren't, they take responsibility for their actions and then move on. Most important, they follow up on their promises in the first place so that they don't have any reason to fabricate excuses. If you want to succeed, you have to make excuses unacceptable. Eventually, your goal should be to rarely have a need to make excuses. Once you're committed to making your body over, you'll be so self-disciplined that you'll make good on your promises—there will be no reason to have to try to justify your bad behavior because it won't exist. First, though, you need to look at the excuses you're throwing out now, own up to the real reasons for your actions, and contemplate ways you can change.

Giving Up Easily: Do setbacks routinely knock you off course?

Life is full of setbacks, but some people don't see them for what they really are: temporary, not permanent, hindrances. What happens to you when the gains you made in an area—be it losing weight, mastering a sport or hobby, succeeding on the job—either stagnate or reverse? Do you usually just give up? Do you feel discouraged and angry? How much of a perfectionist are you? Do you think that anything that can't be done perfectly shouldn't be done at all?

I think it's fair to say that nobody who has succeeded in any area of life has made it without experiencing setbacks. If you're disheartened by even small disappointments, you're going to find it difficult to reach your goals. Have you already let setbacks deter you in the past? And—think carefully here—was the setback really such a failure? What makes you feel as though you have to be perfect or that you won't be able to recover from a defeat? Now think about instances when you *didn't* let setbacks stop you from reaching your goal. When have you and when haven't you persevered, and what was the difference between the two experiences?

If you haven't noticed by now that life is a roller coaster, then you haven't been paying attention. You're going to have ups and downs—everybody does—and your success is going to hinge on how well you weather the downs. Many people I know use setbacks to let themselves off the hook. Consciously or unconsciously, they secretly want the opportunity to get out of the hard work of change or to confirm that they weren't meant to achieve what they set out to do. Sometimes these are hard traits to recognize in yourself. It's really important to acknowledge how you have dealt with disappointments in the past and to dig deep to understand why you let them knock you off course.

Don't be someone who lets setbacks invalidate all your previous efforts and keep you from making ongoing attempts to change your life. Don't use them as an excuse to give up. Not being able to sweep minor failures under the carpet and get on with life is a major reason for ultimate failure. Don't give in to the little failures—they'll just turn into big ones. Keep your focus on the progress you've made. Be prepared to experience setbacks, to acknowledge them, and then to move on.

Part of this is being realistic. Know, for instance, that if one night you slip up and eat a piece of cake, you're not going to weigh three pounds more the next day. More important, there's no reason not to get back on track. Setbacks can be depressing, but don't use the disappointment you're feeling as a justification for overeating and forgoing exercise. Successful people have an ability to roll with the punches, a skill you're going to need to master if you too hope to succeed. Some people come by the skill naturally, but others have to develop it, and you can do that by focusing on the truth: setbacks are bumps in the road; they are not the *end* of the road.

Immediate Gratification: Are you impatient if you don't see results right away? Do you opt for what feels good now over what will feel good later?

If there is a litmus test for success at weight loss, getting fit, and changing your health profile, it's whether you constantly need immediate gratification. People who can defer gratification usually lose weight and become healthy and fit; those who live for immediate gratification usually don't. If you can't master the urge to satisfy yourself in the short term, you're going to have a long, hard road in front of you.

Impatience is rampant these days, and it's not hard to see why. We live in a "fast" society: everything from information on the Internet to food comes to us quickly—more quickly than we might even have imagined just a few short years ago. It's no wonder, then, that most people are intolerant of anything short of immediate gratification. But are you chronically impatient? Does your desire to have everything *right now* extend to all aspects of your life? Are you anxious to be on the next rung of your career ladder when you've just started your new job? Do you want your financial investments to pay off overnight? Do you expect to be instantaneously accomplished at any skill, from tennis to painting, you take on yourself to learn? When it comes to your body, do you want to participate in an exercise class, go home, and see a different body in the mirror? Do you want to eat less on one day and weigh less the very next?

Getting what you want right now doesn't jibe with achieving weight loss; you must be willing to delay gratification. Many an immediate gratification junkie has given up because he or she didn't see change right away. These people are also prone to opting for what makes them happy in the short term over what will make them happy in the long term. How many times have you chosen a piece of cake for dessert because it offers instant fulfillment over the delayed satisfaction of having a thinner, healthier body? How many times have you skipped a workout to sleep late now, the prospect of being fitter later be damned? You can probably detect this same kind of behavior in other areas. Was there a time, for instance, when you bought yourself a new outfit instead of tucking the money away towards vacation? Are there times when, to the contrary, you've waited to get the things you want? How did that feel, and can you see yourself doing it again?

Deflecting temptation and delaying satisfaction aren't easy. But succeeding at making yourself over depends on your ability to delay gratification, to pass on temptations by looking and striving toward the future. This is one of the hardest parts, if not *the* hardest, of making yourself over. You have to be willing to make sacrifices. You can't (literally and figuratively) have your cake and eat it, too.

But if you've lived your life giving in to the need for immediate satisfaction, how do you change? One thing that helps is to constantly remind yourself of what your goals are and how important they are to you. When temptation strikes during this 12-week program (and it will!), picture yourself accomplishing what you've set out to and reflect on how gratifying it will be if you can just get past the moment of temptation. (And often it *is* just a moment—sometimes if you just wait for a minute or two instead of acting right away, the desire will pass.) It can also help to surround yourself with reminders of what you want to achieve: an article of clothing you hope to fit into one day; pictures of yourself at a weight you aim to return to; entry blanks for 5K or 10K runs you want to participate in; pamphlets for hiking or biking trips you'd like to go on when you're fit enough. Anytime you're tempted to miss an exercise session or eat something you know isn't good for you, use these talismans to remind you of your goals. You might even try writing down what you're giving up and what, in the future, you'll get in return. Seeing it in black and white may make your choice much clearer.

Use imagery, too. When you're standing in front of the refrigerator deciding whether or not to dive into the leftovers from dinner, conjure up images of yourself reaching your goal. Keep that vision in your mind's eye, and it will help you get through tough times.

Focus on the positive things that are happening. Too often people have their eyes only on the main prize—a fitter body—when there are many smaller prizes to be had as well. As you get fitter, do you find yourself feeling better? Sleeping better? Do you have the energy to do things, such as playing with your kids, that you weren't able to do before? Have you discovered that you have the strength to lift weights? Have you become fit enough to increase your level of aerobic exercise? These are all important accomplishments that signal that you are becoming healthier—and that really should be your number one goal. Good health is the ultimate reward.

Here is something else that I think will eventually get you through times of temptation: habit. As you get going on this program, you will develop new, healthier habits. If you show some strength—and this, obviously, is the most challenging part—pretty soon your need for immediate gratification will subside as your healthy habits take over. Sloughing off exercise will be less of a temptation when you're in the habit of working out. Likewise, eating foods that you know aren't healthful will be less alluring when you are used to consuming more nutritious foods. I'm not saying that temptation ever completely goes away, but if you can avoid caving in early on, it does get easier as you go along.

What I'm asking you to do here is to think differently about the fleeting pleasure of giving into temptation. Small sacrifices now will have a big payoff later. Stay focused on your goal of making your body over, and you'll be less prone to giving in to immediate gratification.

Laying Blame: Do you always find someone or something else to blame for your actions?

The easiest way to let yourself off the hook for something you're ashamed of or embarrassed about is to lay blame elsewhere. The recipient of your blame might be your job, your family, some nebulous force in the universe—it doesn't really matter. If you're not taking responsibility for your own actions or failings, you are never going to be able to make changes and stick with them.

In my line of work, I see a lot of blamers. Blamers don't feel as though they're in control of their own life, and, like excuse makers, they're always trying to justify their actions. Think a minute about your obligations to others and whether they keep you from fulfilling your obligations to yourself. Do you devote the time you could be exercising to your work instead? Do you let your family's food needs take precedence over your own? There's no doubt that work and family should be priorities, but why can't your own needs also be satisfied? Isn't there a happy medium that you may be overlooking? Contemplate the family and work situations that have led you to give up on your goals. Be honest about whether you used them as excuses or they were legitimate. Say, for instance, that you give up morning walks because they didn't give you enough time to get the kids ready for school. Okay, so why couldn't you get up a half hour earlier or get a walk in later in the day? These are the kinds of things I want you to think about as you consider where you're laying the blame for your behavior.

What worthwhile thing have you accomplished in your life? Did you do so by making it a top priority? Chances are the answer is yes. Life just doesn't work any other way. It follows, then, that if you're going to change your life, *you* have to be among your top priorities.

That means that if you don't accomplish what you planned to, *you* are to blame—not anyone or anything else.

Reshuffling your life to put health and fitness goals front and center can be unsettling. But look at it this way: you are going to be a much better friend, spouse, significant other, parent, employee, employer—whichever role(s) you play in daily life—if you are happy and healthy. Maybe the airline metaphor is overused, but let me throw it out there anyway. There's a reason why, in case of emergency, the flight attendants ask you to first place the oxygen mask over your own face before assisting children: you're not going to do them any good if you can't breathe yourself! The same is true when it comes to your health: though you may think you are sacrificing your own goals for others, in fact, you are doing them a disservice by not being the best you can be. If you stay on track, your relationships with others will benefit tremendously, and you will also be setting a good example for people you care about and who care about you. This is especially important if you are a parent. Kids mimic their parents' behavior, and, especially in this age of increasing childhood obesity, it's essential to present them with good role models.

I know what you may be thinking: Reprioritizing is easier said than done! How can I reorder my work or family obligations? If you think creatively, there is always a way. You may have to be more efficient in your other responsibilities; you may have to let some things go and concede that, say, not everything in your house will be put away perfectly or that you will have to say no to covering for a coworker.

One woman who shared her makeover story with me for my Web site faced this problem. Her family protested when she stopped bringing junk food into the house, but when she stood her ground, they eventually came around. "I have a family history of diabetes, and not only did I not want that for myself, I didn't want it for my children or husband," she said. "Now I keep bags of oranges and apples and granola and flavored water in the house instead of chips and soda. The whole family has gotten healthier, and my husband has lost weight, too. At first I got a few frowns, but it's better now—and there is still room for treats in our lives. It's just that now we go out and get ice cream on occasion instead of always keeping a gallon of ice cream in the freezer."

When you think about your obligations to others, be certain that you aren't using those responsibilities as an excuse to let yourself off the hook. If you're just being lazy or avoiding the unpleasant, be honest about it. You're never going to get to the next step if you don't face up to the real reasons why you've failed in the past.

Making Her Health a Priority
Shawn's Story

Many women continue to carry some "baby weight" after they have a child. Multiply it by five—I am the mother of five children, ages 3 to 14—and you can see my predicament. After giving birth to my last child, I found that I weighed 421 pounds.

It may sound surprising, but I had never tried diets or exercise before. Three years ago, though, I was rummaging through a used-book sale and I came upon Bob and Oprah's book *Make the Connection*. I found that the book spoke to me. I looked through it and thought to myself, "I could really do this."

The book stresses that you really have to have a plan and that you should chart your food and water intake as well as everything about your exercise. Keeping a journal is something I still do today. At the end of the week, I look over what I've done and think about what I could have done better. I might, for instance, see that I ate a bran muffin for breakfast, which sounded healthy at the time but, upon reflection, I know deep down has too many calories. Next week, the bran muffin will be out.

So far, I have lost 140 pounds and while I'm not at my goal weight yet, I am continuing to work toward it. And my life has changed drastically. I have so much more energy, am a much more active person, and am eating much more healthfully—as is everyone else in my family.

One of the best steps I took was to follow Bob's advice to

have an eating cutoff time three hours before bedtime. The first month that I started the program, I didn't really see any weight loss, but as soon as I instituted that rule, I lost three pounds. That's probably because I was a big-time night eater. I would get up at three in the morning and eat a big bowl of Lucky Charms or Sugar Pops with full-fat milk. Now I'm rarely hungry enough to eat after my cutoff time, and when I am I know it's because I haven't eaten well during the day.

Changing my eating habits was a gradual process because not only did I have to alter my habits, I had to wean my kids off some of the foods we typically had in the house. So I did things like replace Froot Loops with Cheerios, and once the kids got used to it, they were perfectly happy. I stopped buying potato chips and started sneaking healthy foods like brown rice and beans into casseroles. I bought everyone in the household his and her own water bottle. I found that if there are no other options, they'll eat and drink what's there. If they put up a fuss, I just tell them, "This is for my health."

I began the exercise part of my program by walking. At first it was all I was able to do. Once I got up to speed, I joined a gym, and now I do a variety of different cardiovascular exercises. I work out on the elliptical trainer, ride the stationary bike, and walk on the treadmill. Once I started weight training, more inches came off. My weight actually went up a little, but I came down in body fat. I now go to the gym six days a week and strength train two to three times weekly.

When you have five children, it's not easy to fit in exercise, but I made it a priority. I decided that I was going to give myself permission to put myself first, because at the end of the day I'm able to do a lot more for other people when I'm also doing something for myself. So even when I was working, I made sure that I had some time to exercise. I schedule the kids' activities around the time I go to the gym or walk. I tell them, "This is the time I have available to take you places," and it seems to work out. They often walk with me, although they could keep up with me better in the beginning. Now that I walk faster, it's a little harder for them.

My being active has benefited my children. Now I have the energy to stay up in the evenings and watch the boys play basketball. We hike and backpack, and I play with the kids at the playground. Once I was on the swing, and a woman came up and asked me if I wasn't embarrassed to be on the swing because I was so heavy. Another time I was Rollerblading, and some people worried about what they would do if I fell. Would they have to pick me up? Despite the hurtful things that people say, I decided I was not going to just sit on a park bench and watch my children. My daughter jogs and one day I'd like to be able to run with her and to help my boys with soccer.

I want to be part of my kids' lives. I want my children to learn to be healthy and to question what's in the things they're eating. I do things like instead of ordering a take-out pizza, I make my own with whole wheat crust, lots of veggies, and lean Canadian bacon on top. My kids love it and have learned that healthy food can taste good, too.

One of the hard things about losing weight when you have a lot to lose is that people might not notice it at first. I lost about 70 pounds before people started noticing. And even if the numbers on the scale are dropping, they never feel like they're going low enough. So I had to learn to look for other ways to measure my success. One of them was my dress size. When I was a size 32 dress, I bought a 24, and now wear that dress. I'm going to buy myself a size 16 bathing suit this year in anticipation of where I'll be next summer. I also measure myself, because inches lost tell part of the story too. I still weigh myself, but only about once a month.

I have found that the more I stick to my program, the more committed I become. But before you become committed, I think you have to find a reason for doing what you're going to do. My reason was and still is simple: I want to be a good mom to my kids!

Losing weight has changed my life in ways that I would never have imagined. For example, people are starting to ask me how I've lost weight, and I tell them my story, which has helped me to make new friends—being so heavy had tended to make me shy away from people in the past. I also never used to go to the movies because I couldn't fit into the seat, but recently I went with my kids. It was the first time in their lives that we all went to the movies as a family. All along they thought I was crying because of the movie, but I was really crying because I realized that I am now able to do "normal things" like sitting in a booth at a restaurant as well.

I think my relationship with my husband has also improved. I notice that I don't put myself down and that I accept the blame when things aren't going right. I have also accepted the fact that I have made some bad choices, not just in the foods I used to buy but in the way I spent money and paid the bills. I had bad habits when it came to those things, and now I budget our money and have learned to spend wisely. I used to buy things to comfort myself and to make myself feel better—things like lotions and body sprays and perfumes. But now I am confident enough to say I am worth it. I am worth being happy, and I don't need those things to make me happy. Just by living my life I am happy, and by being productive I am making a difference in my life and in the lives of my children. Most people think that loving yourself is a given, but I never did. I see that I had no self-love because I wouldn't take care of myself. Now, though, I'm learning to love and accept myself with all my assets and all my flaws as well.

Enabling Saboteurs: Do you let other people prevent you from succeeding?

You just read about how family and other people close to you can sometimes interfere with the process of change. Sometimes, the problem is not so much that you're laying the blame on other people but that you are allowing other people to dictate the choices you make. Often people sabotage those they love. It may be, for instance, that you have a significant other who is not only unsupportive of your goals but who actively tries to interfere with them by making derogatory remarks, refusing to alter his or her schedule to help you make time for exercise, acting hurt or angry if you want him or her to change the type of food they make for you, even "not letting" you do things such as joining a gym or participating in a walking group. These are just some of things saboteurs do, sometimes unconsciously, although sometimes with full awareness.

And why, subconsciously or not, do they do it at all? Sometimes it can be jealousy—they don't want you to become more attractive to other people, or if they lack willpower of their own, they're envious of your determination. Some people feel threatened by having someone close to them change because it forces them to look at their own situation and challenges them to do something about it. Some people are just used to exercising control over what their significant other does and doesn't do. Generally, what drives all of these things is fear: they are afraid of being left behind. You are improving yourself, which may cause them either to fear that you will elevate yourself right out of their sphere of influence or to fear that you will become "better" than they are because they haven't also done what they need to do to change.

Look at your own situation and think about it. Do you feel anxious when trying to cut calories or increase your exercise because you know that you're going to hear some smart remarks from—or even experience the anger of—your friends or family? Do friends or other people close to you try to entice you to eat foods that are fattening or to skip your workouts and go out to dinner instead? Do they tell stories about others who have tried to make healthful changes and failed? Open up your ears and eyes to see what's really going on.

You don't live alone in a cave; I know your family and social relationships are very important to you. But you have to take a look at those relationships for what they are. If someone is not being supportive of you or is actually trying to sabotage your efforts to lose weight and improve your health, that relationship needs to change. The best-case scenario is to get that person on board not only to support and encourage you to but to join you in getting healthy. You may find however, that you will have to reevaluate that relationship. Here's a story that illustrates the best-case scenario.

Mutual Support
Dee and James's Story

Dee: I am five feet, two inches and used to wear a size 20. I had to shed about 60 pounds to reach my goal. Looking back, I realize that though I lost all that weight in about six months, it took about 12 years for me to find the will to change my lifestyle and my way of eating. All that time I had been dieting off and on, losing and gaining but never getting anywhere. I always wanted to be able to say "I did it!" I wanted to experience the joy. I wanted to be who I am now, wearing size 10. I had prayed for it for years. I had prayed alone, I had prayed with my husband. And then one day I saw Bob's article in *O* magazine, and it all came together. I said to myself, "This time I will be able to do it." I filled out the form and mailed it to Bob and Oprah.

It would not have happened without my husband's support. I told him that this was a turning point in my life—that I had signed a Contract with Myself and that I needed him to help me keep my word. I asked him to play a role in my diet for six months. I asked him not to bring any food into the house that wasn't on my diet. No soft drinks, no sweets, no junk-food snacks, no fried chicken. James is a very good man. We have been married 18 years. He agreed on the spot to help me.

James: In the past, when Dee was dieting I didn't participate. She had tried several plans, none of them with lasting results. But this time I could tell it was different. She was serious. She explained that it would increase her chance of success if I followed the diet with her. I didn't think much about it. "Sure," I said, "I'll do it with you!"

Maybe it was my male ego, but I didn't think that I had to lose that much weight. I was 210 pounds at the time, with a 38-inch waist, and pretty confident about my looks. But then the first week, I lost about eight pounds, my clothes got looser, and I felt better. "Wow," I thought, "I have to keep doing this thing!" I lost 35 pounds, and now I have a 32-inch waist. I am in it for the long run.

Dee: The new eating plan was simple. A friend of ours who had lost a lot of weight had given it to me. We had to eliminate sugar, salt, bread, and soft drinks. We also had to give up fried food. We are from the South, natives of Tennessee, and have lived in Memphis, Nashville, and now Atlanta. Fried food is a tradition with us. We had to learn a completely different way of cooking. We began to grill fish, chicken, and beef.

James: We had a gas grill on our porch. We fired it up! We grilled in the rain. We grilled in winter. We grilled twice a day. We grilled food in advance and then put it in the freezer. It was great. And I was happy to help Dee prepare meals and be so much part of the whole process. Not to mention that the cleaning up afterward was much simpler than when she was cooking on a stove!

Dee: We removed all the products that would cause us to gain weight or tempt us to eat when we were not hungry. I stopped buying oil, quite a switch for me! I also stopped using a lot of butter—I used to use so much in mashed potatoes and on the green vegetables. We got rid of the salt and instead learned to cook with herbs, spices, and garlic powder. We filled our refrigerator and pantry with healthy snacks such as applesauce, fresh pineapple chunks, and sugar-free Jell-O.

I realized that changing one's ways is a question of discipline. Without it, no one can give up old habits or learn new techniques. In general, I stopped thinking about taste and instead focused on the foods' benefits to my health and weight.

We told our teenage children that if they wanted to eat sweets or unhealthy food, they would have to buy their own single servings or eat at the mall. They agreed. Sometimes my son teases me and tells me that he loved me just as much when I was my fat, warm, and cuddly self!

Members of our extended family are supportive as well. At the beginning they weren't sure, but now they know that I mean it when I say that I don't eat fried food anymore. At the last family gathering, they grilled food instead of frying it. I was very impressed.

James: Our exercise routine has been the same for the last 20 years. Dee and I exercise on the treadmill at home for about 30 minutes a day at least five days a week. Maybe that's why, at our age and in spite of the excess weight we have carried around all these years, we have maintained good health—we have good blood pressure, low cholesterol, and are not diabetic. I am 40 and Dee is 42, but we feel and look years younger since we changed our diet and dropped all those pounds.

Together, we have relearned how to eat. Now we pray every night out of gratitude. Our prayers keep us focused and motivated.

Dee had it pretty easy with James. She asked him to be supportive, and he didn't hesitate to jump on her bandwagon. Some of you might not have it so easy, but you still need to take that first step, which is to ask your partner, family, and/or friends to help you out. Let them know that you are serious about your commitment to change, then *show* them you are serious about change through your actions. Ultimately, you can really strengthen your relationships by starting a dialogue about your needs and asserting your independence. Remember, though, that whether your friends and family are supportive or not, the buck still stops with you. They may make it more difficult for you to accomplish your goals, but if you really want to do so, no one can stop you from achieving them.

If encouragement and assistance aren't forthcoming, you'll need to do some serious thinking about whether you want to continue to have a relationship with the person or persons who are being unsupportive. In some cases, you may need to move on. Many people have found that in fact the real change they needed to make was not what they ate for dinner, but something much larger: they needed to change or let go of a relationship, and once they did, making changes in their health-related behavior came a lot more easily. (See Angela's story on page 68.)

Procrastination: Do you never do today what you can put off till tomorrow?

Everybody puts things off once in a while, but chronic procrastinators put off just about everything. The trouble is, they often put off things so long that they never get around to doing them at all. How well does this describe you? If you are a procrastinator, why do you let things slide? Is it laziness, or is it fear of change? Replay some of the times when you've procrastinated, then ask yourself what stood in your way. It's really crucial that you be honest here because in order to succeed you have to break the cycle of procrastination, and to do that you have to understand why you drag your feet all the time. Dig down deep on this one: Are you simply avoiding the discomfort of making healthy changes, or are you worried that your life will change in ways that you may not be able to cope with?

I wish we had another word for lazy. The "L" word is just about the worst thing you can label someone in this society; no one likes to be called lazy. But I'm not talking about always-sitting-in-a-La-Z-Boy-chair-with-a-mai-tai kind of lazy, I'm talking about emotional laziness (okay, and when it comes to exercise, some physical laziness, too). You know things need to change, but you don't make the effort. You're always putting things off and taking the easy way out. Letting yourself off the hook. That's the kind of lazy I'm talking about.

If laziness is behind your procrastination, you have to change—*now*. What's often overlooked about procrastination is what accompanies it: feelings of guilt and anger at oneself. So take the bull by the horns and get going. Start a cycle of positive momentum by taking small steps toward your goals each day and feeling good about each of those steps that you take. Make a list of all the things you need to get you going—whether it be arranging for child care so you can exercise, joining a gym, stocking your kitchen with healthful foods, or visiting a farmers' market. Write down a start date for each, and then stick to that calendar.

If laziness is not your problem, is it fear? What are you afraid of? Change takes you from your comfort zone into the unknown, so it's not unusual to feel anxious. But to make your body over, you must be willing to live outside your comfort zone. That's a trait all of the successful folks you're reading about possess: they're brave.

Fear of change stops lots of people in their tracks. People who have this fear sometimes even breathe a sigh of relief when they encounter a setback because it allows them to go back to their old ways. But what is it that's so scary? For some people it's actually fear of success. Being overweight helps make many people feel as if they are invisible. Losing weight literally uncovers them, ending or at least reducing their self-imposed protection from everyday life. Often they seek ways to sabotage themselves so that they can return to the safety their excess weight provides. Or they just procrastinate and don't start at all.

If this is you, take heart. When you do find the courage to risk change and experience it in small doses, at your own rate, you'll be in for wonderful life changes. You can't know what the water is like until you put a toe in. So start small, but *do* start, and see where it leads. There aren't many people who can say that losing weight has been detrimental to their life. Sure, you will have adjustments to make and you will have to deal with people complimenting you and paying attention to you in admiring ways. Nice as that is, it can also make you wonder why they weren't paying attention to you before. It's a good question, but the answer doesn't really matter (and is best left to social scientists). What matters in the end is that by making your body over, you will be a healthier and—odds are—happier person. Ask yourself what you would leave behind if you lost weight. Probably nothing worth holding on to. Fear is not always an easy thing to overcome, but once you do, your life will change for the better.

Dwelling in the Past: Do you blame your current life on something that happened a long time ago?

There's no doubt that our past shapes us in fundamental ways. Yet none of us has to be defined by what happened in our formative years. By asking if you're dwelling in the past, I'm asking if you can't let go of long-ago incidents and relationships that affected you deeply. Has your self-image been shaped by earlier events to such a degree that it's hindering your future? How attached are you to the present? Do you feel paralyzed because you can't see yourself any other way than the way you are now?

If you answered yes to any of these questions, you need to take some time and revisit the past. It may cause you discomfort or even pain, I know, but it's an essential part of the truth-telling process. Dredge up any memories that have to do with how you feel about your body. It may be related to how members of your family or those close to you treated you. For instance, some people who were taunted for being fat by parents or siblings end up staying that way because they use food to soothe away the pain of being ridiculed. It could be some type of abuse you were subject to, either physical or emotional, that's caused you to hide behind your weight. Maybe your problem has more to do with your familial approach to food. Many families equate food with love, and to reject food is to reject love. As you reflect, think about how you've learned to cope with any painful issues, incidents, or relationships. They may hold the key to why you're holding on to being overweight.

The past is past. It's time to start living in the present and making changes that will enhance your future. While certainly what happened long ago has influenced your life, that's no excuse for using it as a crutch. Successful people break the cycle of self-abuse that comes from clinging to unpleasant or even horrible experiences. Show some strength and stop blaming events, family, significant others, anyone or anything else for your eating and exercise habits. You can't change the past, but you can change how you deal with it. *Join life.* Life has both pleasures and pain, and you learn from both. If you're ready to do that, you're ready to begin making your body over.

Asking the Big Questions
Jeff's Story

Sometimes it takes a crisis to bring your life into focus. I was 39 years old and had ended up in the hospital in critical condition, my body overcome by diabetes. I'm a big man, six feet two, but the 310 pounds I was carrying was taking a big toll on both my body and my mind.

When the fog of that episode began to lift, I had to ask myself why I wasn't achieving what I desired. It wasn't as if I didn't try to be healthy, but I had a lot of the wrong ideas about things. I was lifting weights six times a week and eating lots of hamburgers and steaks. I'd work out for two hours and then go eat fried chicken, figuring that I was exercising the calories away. I tried different diets and even tried visualizing myself at a healthy weight, but the pounds kept piling on month after month.

When I was 18, I was applying for a summer job when I was approached by Oprah, who happened to be in the same place that day. She must have sensed my depression, because she offered some kind words. She told me that I could be whatever I wanted to be, and she made me promise I wouldn't give up. Just to be kind back, I agreed.

Twenty-two years later, when my struggle with weight brought me to the place where I had no choice but to maintain a healthier diet, there Oprah was again. This time, she was eighty-five pounds lighter and had kept the weight off for more than two years with help of Bob Greene. Part of my reeducation on eating was found in *Make the Connection* by Bob and Oprah. Reading through Oprah's stories about her own weight loss battles along with the encouragement and advice she and Bob provided helped walk me toward a healthier and happier existence.

Most important, I asked myself, "Why am I here, and how can I battle what I cannot see?" The answer came to me through keeping a daily journal. It allowed me to ask myself powerful and, at times, painful questions. Answering those questions became my private therapy session, helping me to take a good hard look at what I was truly battling. One of the things that I realized was that because of the abuse I'd suffered as a child I was trying to make myself big so no one could take advantage of me ever again. Not surprisingly, I was not succeeding at trying to be big and lose weight at the same time.

Since I made that connection, I have become 30 pounds lighter and much healthier. For the first time I realized what I was doing, and I was able to let it all go. I've learned to eat more nutritiously, and even though I sometimes eat foods I know I shouldn't, I have been able to maintain a healthier diet. I've gone from taking insulin three times a day to twice a week. I do cardiovascular exercise every day, generally doing 20 to 30 minutes in the morning and 30 minutes to an hour in the evenings. In the summer and spring I walk, and in the winter and fall I do tae bo. I also work out on the treadmill and elliptical machine and do wind sprints on the track. I've cut back my weight training to one day a week (for some reason lifting causes my blood sugar to rise). I have 20 more pounds to go before I achieve the body I've been visualizing, but I'm making progress.

Since dropping the weight, I no longer suffer from nagging back pain, shortness of breath, or trying to find clothes that fit (I can now tuck my shirt in and see my feet while standing up). I feel that I can achieve anything I set my mind to, and, released from the prison of fear and failure, I am free to create the life I want. I am no longer affected by life; life is now affected by me. The promise I made years ago not to give up has been fulfilled.

The Second Cornerstone: Responsibility

I once worked with a client who was a tremendously honest person. He was willing to own up to all his weaknesses, which included a tendency to try to cut corners and a strong attachment to immediate gratification. But while he was willing to own up to these shortcomings, he wasn't willing to *own* them—and those are two different things. "That's just the way I am," he would say, as if he were a robot who had been programmed, with no will of his own. He could swallow the notion that his actions were detrimental to his health and weight loss goals, but not the notion that he could change those actions. Taking responsibility wasn't in his realm of possibilities.

Until one day it was. After his wife asked him for a divorce, he really reflected on his behavior, realized it was his responsibility to change it, and decided that he would. Now he's remarried, has money in the bank (he was always broke before), and very happy. The divorce motivated him to change his core behavior. As a result, everything else in his life improved too.

Leveling with yourself is just the first step to building a sound emotional foundation. But successful people don't just tell the truth, they also take responsibility for it. They vow to change and make good on that promise. Saying "That's just the way I am, and I'll have to work around it" won't get you anywhere. Saying "That's how I *used* to be, but I'm not going to be that person anymore" will.

The real challenge you have ahead of you is to change things about you that may be central to your personality. To make that possible, you need to stop pointing to external reasons for the state of your weight and your health. The way you were brought up, your significant other, the stress of your job or parenting duties—none of these things is to blame for your behavior. You can no longer fall back on saying "My mother did this to me," "My husband and kids won't eat that," "My boss demands this and that." It's simply not going to wash anymore. You've got to look at the truth about *you* and stop blaming your life on outside factors. Nor can you put the blame on a world filled with endless temptations (so many wonderful things to eat, so many other things to do besides exercise). The responsibility is yours and yours alone. It all comes down to you. You are in control of your actions and, likewise, in control of making over your body. The people I know who've *changed* their lives *took charge* of their lives. Ask yourself: What kind of life do you want? Define it, work for it, seize it.

Dean, whose story you're about to read, is a perfect example. Dean is a young woman who has had such bad luck that she could easily have laid the blame for her weight problem at fate's feet. Instead, one day she woke up to the fact that she had to take responsibility for her behavior. Today, she has the body to prove that seizing control of your life will set you on the road to success.

I Am Not a Victim
Dean's Story

My journey began on my thirty-second birthday in June 2002. My husband and family had given me a surprise party. It was a joyous occasion—until I saw myself on a video a friend took of the party. I was so disgusted with how incredibly huge and jiggly my body was that I teared up and wanted to run out of the room to hide. Right then I knew for sure that I had to make a big change.

At the time I was a size 16 and was carrying 190 pounds on a five foot, two inch frame. At one point I had even been a size 20 and weighed 215 pounds. Today, I have lost 105 pounds and wear a size 6. Although I still have a little weight to lose, my skin is now firm and my muscles are toned. But to get from there to here turned out to be a physical and emotional rollercoaster ride.

After that fateful birthday, I bought the Atkins diet book and began to read it. I felt as though Dr. Atkins was describing me, and I started the program the very next day. I felt that dieting would be the solution since exercise was difficult; I have fibromyalgia, an incurable chronic pain syndrome that leaves me weak, fatigued, and sore from head to toe.

Still, I bought some yoga and Pilates tapes and began to work out in front of the television while my two older boys were in school. Even though I had to take it slowly, I lost 10 pounds in two weeks.

My health, unfortunately, got in the way. First it was female problems—heavy bleeding, cramping, pain—and it became apparent that I needed a hysterectomy. A date was set for surgery, but two days before the operation, my health insurance company denied my claim. By August, I had to have an emergency D & C, but it didn't solve the problem. I was still bleeding and emotionally drained, so much so that one day I fell apart, sobbing uncontrollably. I literally dropped to my knees to pray and ask God to please give me the strength I needed to lose weight and feel good about myself. I was so sick of being sick!

Before I go on, I want to make it clear that I am not a victim. In fact, I come from a long line of strong women. My grandmother and my mother are my heroes. They taught me to "dream big and do bigger." All through my ordeal, I remembered their example. Giving up was never an option. As my grams used to say, "With perseverance, even the snail made it to the ark."

My real problem is not obesity per se. Since childhood I would denigrate myself and punish myself for things I had no control over. I would medicate myself with food instead of dealing with my low self-esteem. As a child, I blamed myself for the divorce of my parents, feeling that I had failed them somehow. I was present when my twin sister died in a freak accident when we were only six years old. From then on, I thought that I deserved all the cruelty I was to endure, including being sexually molested between the ages of seven and nine.

One day I hit rock bottom. I wept for my traumatic childhood. I wept for my difficult pregnancies and births. I wept for being diagnosed with fibromyalgia and all that goes with this dreadful disease, including severe depression. Finally, I wept for my most recent loss, the death of my grandmother. Then I decided never to cry myself to sleep again and to change my attitude right then and there. I knew that I had to accept who I was in spite of my imperfections.

I fought the insurance company and won. I recommitted to my new lifestyle of low carbs, no sugar, and exercise six days a week. Whenever I felt down, I thought of my children and my husband. To help them, I would have to help myself. Getting well was the greatest way I could show my love for them.

My surgery dates were again postponed. It actually turned out to be a blessing in disguise, because in the process the doctors discovered bladder disease. Finally, in December 2002, I had the hysterectomy and bladder surgeries.

As I slowly recovered, I went back to yoga and Pilates. By January, I had lost 40 pounds and eleven inches around my waist. One Sunday, I was hurrying down the hall when I tripped and fell flat on my face. You can imagine my surprise when I discovered that my slip had dropped down to my ankles. It wasn't my most graceful moment, but it was a moment of crazy joy!

That's when I took Bob and Oprah's challenge and signed the contract with myself. My goal was to lose the rest of the weight within the next twelve weeks. In hindsight, I am so glad I made that official commitment to myself at that point. It helped me through the last big hurdle.

In early February, doubled over with intense abdominal pain, I was admitted to the hospital. I had to have my gall bladder removed, but when I woke up in recovery, I was told that my appendix had also been removed and a liver biopsy performed. I was in the most excruciating pain I have ever experienced.

I had very serious complications and had to be transferred by ambulance to a hospital in San Francisco, a hundred miles away from where I live. My mother took care of my three boys while I underwent five major surgeries in a nine-week period. That's when I came close to dying—and when I decided I could not give up.

I decided I wasn't going to allow anything to keep me from losing weight. I didn't want to die a fat lady! Every time I thought I could not go on, I looked at a photo of my three precious boys and somehow managed to get through it.

It has been a long and slow recovery. Luckily, I didn't gain any weight in the hospital. I was able to return to my diet and yoga, though Pilates was too strenuous for my condition. Though I will never be cured of fibromyalgia, I am no longer plagued with psychological symptoms. I have energy that I've never known before. I have discovered an inner strength I didn't know I had. Instead of hating myself, I now treat myself the way I would treat my best friend. I have become a better individual, wife, lover, mother, daughter, and friend. I have become nicer to be around, able to laugh more and relax.

Originally, my goal was to be the size (10) and have the health I had when I first got married. To my surprise, through my challenging, yet wonderful journey, I have discovered that I can do even better than my twenty-something-year-old self. I am driven, stronger, more patient, more compassionate, much happier, and even smaller today (size 6) than I have ever been in my life!

Through accountability—and not just wanting health but working hard toward it each day—I feel as if I have been given a second chance, and I am not going to waste one second. I feel comfortable in my own skin, flaws and all, and for the very first time in 34 years I have stopped surviving through each day and actually started to live.

I believe in myself now. I have no more fear of trying new things or taking risks. I can look at myself in the mirror and instead of crying because of what I see look deeper and appreciate all the effort and progress I have made. There are still many days when my illness overwhelms me physically and emotionally, but I no longer have to lug around the extra hundred-plus pounds of me, and that helps make the bad days fewer and farther between.

I have come to realize that just like everyone else I too am entitled to joy. Earning my health is what probably means the most to me. I didn't have plastic surgery or eat special foods; I didn't take a magic pill or find a "quick fix." I exercise and eat healthy meals just as I breathe every second or shower and brush my teeth each day. I put my belief in myself into action and have never looked back.

To sum it all up, I guess I would say that life has become a celebration. For me, finding—no, choosing—better health is remembering who I am and finally living up to the potential God labeled "Dean."

One last thing: If I can do this, anyone can! Please, please, believe in yourself. I think Maya Angelou says it best: "I can be changed by what happens to me, but *I refuse to be reduced by it.*"

I am under no illusion that changing your character or letting go of ideas you've been clinging to for years is an easy task, but I also know that it can be done if you take control of your own life (control, which by the way, you've always had but perhaps just chose not to exercise). There's no shame in admitting that in the past you've acted in ways you're not proud of. What matters is what you're going to do right now and in the future. At this time you stand on the dividing line between the old you and the new you—which way are you going to go?

Taking responsibility might simply mean that you admit that you've been lazy and have chosen the easy way out every time; from now on you're not going to let a distaste for hard work get in your way. Or it might mean that you have to make some difficult decisions. If, for instance, you are in a rocky or even demoralizing relationship that's affected your ability to take good care of yourself, then you have to ask yourself what you can do to improve or perhaps even end the relationship. If you have been burying the pain of something terrible that happened long ago under the weight of excess pounds, you need to make a decision about how you can put the past behind you. Maybe you will need to seek professional help to help you deal with the pain. However you choose to approach it, your goal should be to get to a place where you're able to stop blaming the past for your present woes. Free yourself from what's been dragging you down, and you'll have the ability to move on.

Essentially, what I am asking you to do is to take hold of your life—to accept that you've messed up or that you just haven't run your life in an effective manner. Coming to a crossroads can be paralyzing, but I know that it's possible for anyone who really wants to make himself or herself over to get onto the right path. Yes, this is the hand you've been dealt, but you're going to reshuffle the deck and deal yourself a winning hand. Take responsibility for the past and the future, and you'll succeed.

The Third Cornerstone: Commitment

You don't have to look far within our society to see that commitments are no longer as sacred as they once were. It's almost as though not honoring a commitment has become socially acceptable. How often do people make others wait, break dates, not show up, go back on offers to help? It's epidemic.

What does this have to do with weight loss? A lot, in my estimation. If you're lax about your commitments in one area of your life, you're a lot more likely to be lax about other vows you make—both to others and to yourself. It's not a far leap from being late for a dinner date to blowing off a workout; in both cases there's a lack of respect at work.

Successful people keep commitments. They show up on time, they don't break dates, and they don't break promises. Their word is their word, and they stand by it. And, most important, they see themselves as deserving of the same respect they give to others. They keep their commitments to themselves just as they keep their commitments to friends, family, and business associates.

That last part is critical. Maybe you're a little put off by the suggestion that you don't keep commitments, because you are meticulous about keeping promises—to other people! But do you keep the promises you make to *yourself*? A classic trait I see among people who struggle with their weight is that they honor all kinds of commitments to others but always forget to put themselves on the list. They want to be considered "a good person," so they do their utmost to devote themselves to others.

That's selfless; however, it can also border on selfishness. Why?

Because you do a disservice to those who care about you by not taking care of yourself. As nice as it is to be seen as a giving person, you also need to pay attention to your own needs. I know many people who are caretakers of others who don't bother to care for themselves; they cringe at the idea of putting themselves first. But ultimately, if you don't, you won't be much use to anyone else either. And let's be honest: if you don't take care of your health, you run the risk of becoming sick or dying prematurely. How will that help your spouse, your children, your friends, and everyone else who loves and needs you?

I'm not telling you to forget your commitments to others and just concentrate on yourself. But you should examine the reasons you allow the needs of others to take precedence over your own. Why does your commitment to care for your family mean that you can't also fulfill the promise you made to yourself to exercise regularly and eat healthfully? Is your commitment to your work such that there is *no* way to take a walk at lunchtime or get in a meal before you get so ravenous that you grab all the wrong foods? There should be a happy medium that allows you to honor every pledge you make.

This is where I pull out the famous contract. If you're familiar with my work from my other books, magazines, or TV, you know that I believe that signing a contract helps make a commitment sacred. It shouldn't really matter if you put a promise into writing or not; I hope that you would keep it even if the promise exists only in your heart and mind. But somehow, putting pen to paper seems to drive home the seriousness of the endeavor.

Dean, whose story you just read, is only one example of someone who signed the contract to help her honor her commitment to herself. She, like many other people who responded when the contract ran in the January 2003 issue of *O, The Oprah Magazine* and the thousands who have signed it in the *Get With the Program!* books, used it to help her stay committed to a program on which she had already embarked. In your case, you may be signing it before you've made any changes— an excellent way to start. As I've said before, you are much more likely to be successful if you begin by really weighing all the issues: Are you being honest about why you're overweight? Have you owned up to your behavior? And most important, are you truly ready to change? When the answer is yes, the contract on page 58 is waiting for you.

It's Never Too Late to Make the Commitment
Alice's Story

As I write this, I have lost 45 pounds of unhealthy body weight. In the course of a year, I went from a dress size 16 to a size 6. It was a long road getting there. I am 75 years old now, but my weight struggles began when I was very young—they used to call me little bear because I was so chubby. As I got older, boys thought of me as a sister, never as a girlfriend. I even went to my school prom by myself. When I was in college I learned a new way to combat weight: bulimia. It made me thin, but it also made me end up in the hospital. Eventually, I met my husband and married. I was slim at the time; however, shortly after the wedding my weight started rising. After three months of marriage I was so plump my mother-in-law thought I was pregnant!

Things reached a new low in July 2002. My husband had died, and I was eating through the pain—gaining weight because I was depressed and depressed because I was gaining weight. Then a couple of things happened that helped pull me out of the rut and set me on my path to weight loss.

I had looked at Bob's books before, but now I really read them carefully and took to heart a lot of what he had to say. One of his ideas is that to lose weight, you have to love yourself, and that was something I realized was missing in my life: I didn't like me. So I started to do what Bob said. I pledged to eat primarily to satisfy my nutritional needs rather than my emotional needs. I ate fresh fruits and vegetables and baked chicken and fish instead of canned foods. I drank two quarts of water a day and stopped drinking sodas. I began walking five miles a day in beautiful Coral Reef Park in Miami. I discovered that I love to walk. In fact, I was losing weight so fast that my doctor advised me to cut back my walking to three miles a day. That's what I do every weekday and sometimes on Saturdays and Sundays, too. The combination of the exercise and the quiet, meditative time makes me feel wonderful, peaceful, and euphoric. I love walking, and I love *me* much more.

The other inspiration I received came from my parish priest. In one of his sermons during Lent, he spoke on the subject of fasting, a spiritual experience I had always flunked. My priest said that if you have any kind of habit that is more powerful than the God within you, then it is your God. That's when it hit me that food was my God. This was the attitude that was making it very difficult for me to lose the pounds I was fighting so hard to get rid of. With the guidance of my family doctor, I was able to fast for Lent. I lost 20 pounds, but it wasn't really about losing the weight. It was about spiritual empowerment. After it was over, I was able to bring my eating habits under control, and I've gone on to eat sensibly.

I have lost weight before, but what's different this time is that the desire comes from within, not without. My whole outlook has changed, and I'm continuing on my road to a healthier lifestyle under the motto "Nothing—not cake, not candy—tastes better than how being healthy and thin feels." I can really feel the difference, too. I used to suffer from arthritis and no longer do. I feel much more energetic, and I like people more. I'm friendlier!

I'm constantly being told, "Alice, you look so young. You look like a teenager!" Ironically, I do feel like the teenager I was in college with the exception that I now have far more transcendent wisdom. Oprah has said that each time you move toward the life you want, you are doing the most important spiritual work. Well, sticking to my own fitness contract is certainly enabling me to do my most important spiritual work.

TOTAL BODY MAKEOVER

Contract with Myself

I, _____, hereby commit to 12 weeks of regular vigorous exercise and to self-control when it comes to my eating. I will be focused on challenging my abilities in the pursuit of elevating my physical performance. In addition, I will not indulge in any alcoholic beverages during the 12-week period regardless of the nature of the temptation. I will also terminate my consumption of all food two to three hours prior to my bedtime. I will endeavor to be conscious of when and why I eat and will, to the best of my ability, eat simply to satisfy my nutritional needs as opposed to my emotional needs. I will also do my best to make healthful food choices.

I realize that this contract is solely with myself and that it carries no rewards, penalties, or punishments other than those associated with the reflection of the strength of my character.

_____day of_____, 20_____

_____(signature)

The Fourth Cornerstone: Inner Strength

For some reason the idea that losing weight requires willpower has gone out of vogue. Instead, the emphasis over the last few years has been on taking the easy way out. Eat more, weigh less! Exercise just ten minutes a day for a better body! Take a pill and lose weight while you sleep! Eat as much steak, butter, and cheese as you want! But in the end, the idea that changing your body is easy is just wishful thinking.

The ability to impose your will to accomplish what you want to do is what separates those who succeed in any area of life from those who don't. You *do* need willpower, no matter what anyone says. Actually, I prefer to call it inner strength, because those words describe where willpower actually comes from. We all have it deep inside of us; whether you choose to use it is up to you.

I believe that one key to inner strength is making conscious decisions. If you're like most people who struggle with their weight, many of your decisions have become rote reactions, not conscious choices. You come home from a stressful day at work, and you have a drink or dig into a bag of chips; it's a habit. A conscious decision would be to choose to go for a walk instead. You go to a favorite restaurant, and you order the fish and chips because it's what you always get. A conscious decision would be to try the broiled fish. Do you automatically take the elevator instead of the stairs, park as close as possible to your destination, always eat dinner an hour before you go to bed at night? All these things matter, and you should be conscious of them.

All my clients get the "ten-second delay" talk. I ask them to take ten seconds to think about their choices before deciding whether they'll give in to fleeting desires or exercise inner strength to combat them. Ten seconds is just long enough for you to make the decision consciously rather than impulsively. By drawing out the time, you may find that you make a different and much healthier choice whether the choice is between grabbing a cup of yogurt or a piece of cake from the refrigerator or between going to the gym in the morning and rolling over and going back to sleep.

As much as a tool like the ten-second delay can help, in order to draw on your inner strength you're going to have to have made some fundamental changes in your thinking. When you've searched your soul for the reasons you haven't succeeded in the past, owned up to your responsibility for your actions, and really committed to making a change, willpower will be second nature. You'll only need to hone it. Think of your inner strength like a biceps muscle: the more you exercise it, the more powerful you'll be.

Preparing to Change

At this early stage of the program, before you really start taking action to make your body over, I'd like you to think about what you ultimately hope to achieve. It's important to think realistically about your body and how much weight you're capable of losing as well as what you hope weight loss will bring to your life. What is your *real* intention, and how will that intention be realized?

If your intention is to be successful because you truly care about yourself—and not because you are trying to please or attract other people—then your chances of success are greatly increased. This goes back to telling the truth, which I discussed earlier in this chapter. Be honest about why you're going on this program so that you can make sure from the start that you are doing it for the right reasons. Losing weight can make you feel better about yourself, but it's not the ultimate key to happiness. Yes, slimming down can improve your self-esteem, but it can't erase painful experiences from your past that you've avoided dealing with. It can give you newfound or renewed confidence, but it can't make an unhealthy relationship you're in disappear. Don't, in other words, put all your emotional eggs into one weight loss basket. Extra pounds may cause unhappiness, but more often they're a *symptom* of unhappiness.

So don't make weight loss more important than it really is. It's only one way to feel good about yourself. It's healthy to have goals that aren't weight loss–related—learning to play an instrument, doing charitable work, mastering another language, growing a garden in your backyard—the more options you have to help you feel accomplished, the better.

Another thing I think it's important to think about is your ultimate body makeover goals. I'm not going to pretend that most people aren't driven by the goal to look more appealing. There's nothing wrong with that. But I also want to make a case for concentrating on how the changes you make will affect both your health and the way you feel. Those benefits of this 12-week program will come a lot sooner than substantial weight loss, and though you won't necessarily see them staring back at you in the mirror, they're not inconsequential. Eating nutritiously and exercising will do you a world of good above and beyond reducing your body size, so don't take those payoffs for granted.

As you prepare for change, also think about how much change you expect to occur. How much weight do you plan to lose? Most important, is it in your biological nature to accomplish that goal? When you see some of the pictures of makeover success stories on my Website (totalbodymakeover.com), you'll see that not everyone worked him- or herself down to a size 2. Those who did had an inherently thin body hiding underneath the excess pounds. Those who didn't get skinny simply may not have skinny genes. I don't have to tell you that we come in all shapes and sizes and that some people's healthy weight is higher than others. The good news is that everybody can attain a healthy weight for him- or herself.

Consider what's really feasible for you. What is your family history? What is your body type? Even if you can whittle your body down to a very small size, ask yourself what you're going to need to do to sustain it. Will you be able to sustain the low calorie intake and hours of exercise that got you there? Your goal should be to adopt changes that you can sustain for the rest of your life. Keep your goal realistic, and you'll succeed.

The Science of Weight Loss: What You Can Expect to Happen

Did you know that your body allows for only about a loss of three pounds of fat per week? Sure, you can lose water and muscle tissue—

that's how quick-fix diets that promise you'll drop a lot of pounds instantly work—but you don't want to. Everyone loses weight at different rates, but in general losing one pound or even a half pound a week means that you are losing in a way that can last. Quick weight loss, though inspiring and satisfying, hardly ever lasts. Slow going is more frustrating but ultimately offers a bigger payoff. In the beginning, you may find that this 12-week program feels like you're rolling a boulder up a hill—lots of work but no payoff—but I promise you, you will reach the top and begin losing at a faster rate.

In the beginning, as you start exercising and ramping up your workouts and as you change your eating habits, the water your body holds on to (or lets go of) will largely dictate your losses—or even gains. As you become more active and drink more water, your muscles will retain water. The primary culprit here is glycogen, a form of carbohydrate that's stored in your muscles and is the main fuel for exercise. The more active you are, the more glycogen your muscles will retain and thus the more water you'll hold on to: Each gram of glycogen stores an additional 2.5 grams of water. What's more, the fitter you become, the more glycogen you store.

This initial water weight gain can be disheartening, but hang in there. Water-weight gain will cover up the body fat losses that you will be experiencing. After a few weeks, you will begin to see fat loss. And the reality is, this is a part of charging up your metabolism, which will ultimately lead to an increase in your fat-burning power.

The initial weeks of this 12-week program will really be a test of your will. You need to trust that you're doing the right thing, even if it doesn't show up right away on the scale. And while we're on the subject of the scale, try not to get too attached to it. I know that it's hard not to check up on how you're doing constantly, but try to weigh yourself no more than one day a week. Concentrate on how you feel and how your clothes fit. Don't be like the kid in the backseat whining "Are we there yet?" Just be patient. You'll reach your destination, and it's going to be great!

2

ULTIMATE FITNESS

WHAT DOES YOUR CALENDAR look like for the next 12 weeks? The Total Body Makeover is going to require a great deal of dedication, so I want you to make sure that you'll have the time and energy to devote to it. If you want to get into the best shape of your life, you're going to have to put the program at the forefront of your agenda. Doing so will be well worth it, and not just because exercise has the power to reshape your body; it can change everything from your cholesterol count to your attitude about life. In fact, many people start out exercising to get a better body only to wind up staying with it because it makes them feel so good. One of the things that I love about being active myself is that there is always room to get fitter and better at whatever activity (or activities) you do. The challenge never ends.

Whether you haven't intentionally worked out since you were in elementary school or already have a pretty solid fitness program in place and just want to ratchet up the intensity, the 12-week Total Body Makeover plan has something to offer you. What's more, it's going to guide you step by step. A lot of what confounds beginners and sometimes even advanced exercisers is how much exercise they need to do and how hard they need to do it. I'll help you determine the level at which you should start and how quickly you should progress. The only thing you have to do is stay committed and follow along.

One thing I want you to understand about this program is that it's intensive for everyone, no matter where they fall on the fitness scale. Beginner, intermediate, advanced—there is a demanding, yet invigorating exercise regimen in store for each of you. Usually, I start clients out on a slower path. I don't, for instance, have beginners start strength training until about week six (here you'll start in week one, and I also bump up the workouts of intermediate and advanced exercisers). But the goal of this program—to get you substantial results in a faster-then-usual amount of time—requires a different strategy. It's still a safe, healthy strategy, and it's not a quick fix. You will see significant changes in your body in a relatively short time, but the program will also put you onto the road to long-term fitness, and that's what really counts.

The fact that condensing the program will allow you to see results sooner than you otherwise might is not the plan's only benefit. I like to think of it as akin to interval training. For those of you who aren't familiar with the term, interval training is a technique athletes use to improve their fitness so that their usual workouts become a lot easier. It involves stepping up the intensity of their workouts for a short time in order to train their bodies to tolerate a higher workload, then backing off and returning to their usual pace. In a sense you'll be doing the same thing: working hard for 12 weeks so that when you return to a maintenance regimen, it will feel easier. Your less intensive workouts will almost feel normal, not as if you're in training. Again, this is what elite athletes do: they alternate periods of intense and more relaxed training.

The beauty of this program is that it accommodates all levels of fitness. From week to week you'll be following a progression that's appropriate for you wherever you are on the fitness continuum—beginner, intermediate, or advanced.

Although this is an intensive program, if you're a beginner, you don't have to worry that you'll be asked to do more than you can handle. The last thing I want to do is turn you off to exercise by making you overdo it at the outset. But by the same token, I'm not going to let you get overly comfortable with an easy little routine. You'll see dramatic changes because you're going to be very active—not to the point of pain but to the point where you're definitely challenged.

To work its magic, exercise has to be demanding; sometimes you may want to quit or just simply not show up. But 99 times out of 100 you're going to feel so good at your workout session's end that you won't regret one minute of it. You'll also love the results. Granted, some people will never like exercise, but they still do it because they feel that the payoff is so great. It's far more common, though, for people—those, that is, who take the time to really develop a solid workout program—to get hooked on exercise. They just don't feel a hundred percent if they're not active.

If you're an intermediate exerciser—someone, that is, who works out regularly for at least a half hour at a stretch—you probably already know what I'm talking about. You just need to up the ante and perhaps add some variety to your routine; this is the plan that's going to help you do it. You're right on the cusp of doing enough exercise to significantly alter your whole physiological makeup; you just need to increase the challenge to your system. Your work here will be to move from active to athletic.

I'm also throwing down the gauntlet to the advanced exerciser. If you've been training long and hard for many years but want even better results, this is your chance to shake things up and challenge your body in new and different ways. Even passionate exercisers can get in a rut. Think of the next 12 weeks as a boot camp to get you ultrafit and open you up to new possibilities.

One of the most meaningful things you can do in life is to rise up to meet a challenge and achieve your goals. That's what I call *living*, engaging all the resources—physical, mental, and spiritual—that are at your disposal and making them work for you. In the end you will change your body, but the real reward—changing how you feel as well as many other aspects of your life that are unrelated to how you look—will be so much more substantial. If you've been holding off accepting the challenge of transforming yourself, you've been holding off on real life. Now's the time to jump in with both feet. I know you'll be glad you did.

The Fitness Building Blocks of This Program

Before you turn to the week-by-week plan that begins on page 168, I want to explain the fitness fundamentals on which the program is based, beginning with the reasons exercise is so critical to a healthy life. Sure, you know exercise is good for you, blah, blah, blah—you've probably heard it all. But I think if you have a greater understanding of what is actually taking place in your body as you work out, you will be all the more motivated to become a regular exerciser or to take the workouts you already do a step further. I want you to be aware, too, that there is exercise and there is exercise: the exercise regimen that health experts tell you will help you live healthier is not necessarily the same as the one that will help you make your body over.

It's not bad to move only as much as needed to reduce your risk of disease and premature death, but it's usually not enough if you want to see impressive aesthetic results. And, truthfully, it's not enough to get optimal health results either. It's the bare minimum. The more exercise you do (within reason—it *is* possible to do too much) the fitter *and* healthier you'll be. And as I said earlier, if you expect to see some solid transformation in 12 weeks, you really have to step up to the plate. So while I'm pleased that anyone who used to spend most of his or her time on the couch now walks for 20 minutes at lunchtime three days a week, that's not going to cut it if your goal is a total body makeover in three months.

No matter what your starting point is (which I'll help you determine on page 76), you have to do more than the bare minimum—and you have to progress significantly. The exercise recipe I consider best for success is analogous to heating milk on the stove. When you heat milk, you need to keep the temperature high enough to allow the milk to warm gradually, but not so high that the milk boils over the sides of the pan and burns. Similarly, you want the amount of exercise you do to put you on a steady path to reaching your goal, but you don't want it to be so hard that you end up burned out, injured, or both. If you find that the workout goals I've mapped out for you each week are just too difficult to accomplish, cut back to a level you can maintain. But remember that this program isn't supposed to be easy. The exercise will get slightly easier once you've conditioned your body.

Discomfort is a funny thing. In most cases, we do our best to avoid it, yet without discomfort you can't make any meaningful fitness gains. This isn't quite the same thing as "no pain, no gain"; that can be a dangerous philosophy in exercise because pain can lead to injury, and with injury, of course, there are no gains. Discomfort, on the other hand, means that you are making a breakthrough. Discomfort informs your body that it needs to be stronger, and the body, through its natural physiology, complies. It's a paradox, but successful people are comfortable with discomfort. They allow themselves to feel it—and to push past it. In an earlier chapter I asked you to do some self-examination that may have been uncomfortable for you, the goal being to let yourself experience this state of uneasiness so that you could end up free of it. It's the same thing here. In short, the fitter you get, the more pleasurable exercise will be.

The type of workouts you'll be doing over the next 12 weeks fall into three categories: functional exercises, strengthening exercises, and aerobic exercise. This is a holistic approach to fitness. Each type of activity creates different benefits, and it's only when you combine them that you can achieve ultimate fitness. And while each type of exercise trains your body in separate ways, they're all pieces of the fitness pie; put them together, and they equal a whole—and a whole new body for you.

Have you ever met a marathon runner who has trouble lifting her kids? Or a body builder who can barely make it on the treadmill for more than five minutes? Although I'm hoping that you will find one or two activities that you truly love doing, it's important not to focus on them to the exclusion of other exercises. If you already have a one-dimensional workout that you're devoted to, now's the time to expand your regimen.

Let me tell you a little more about each of the three types of workouts. Functional exercises improve your flexibility, balance, coordination, and the strength of key muscle groups. Mostly specific strengthening exercises, stretches, and balancing moves, they not only help you perform the strengthening and aerobic portions of your workouts with greater ease, they also make your everyday movements more graceful and efficient.

Strengthening exercises, as their name suggests, make you stronger, though they also have other benefits, including helping to prevent the muscle and bone deterioration that comes with age. They keep your metabolism—the rate at which you burn calories—in high gear. You can strength train with exercise bands and other resistance tools—even your own body weight—but probably the most common type of resistance training involves weights. The beginning exercises here can be done with dumbbells, though as you progress you will also need to use the kind of weight machines found in most gyms.

This program calls for everyone, beginners included, to start strength training in week one. A word of warning, though, to those of you who have never lifted weights before: many people find that strength training increases their appetite. If you're already struggling with your eating habits, this can be problematic, but I think if you know ahead of time that you may experience increased hunger on days when you lift, you'll be better able to cope with it.

The last piece of the puzzle is aerobic exercise. Aerobic (or cardiovascular) workouts, the kind that elevate your heart rate, are the real calorie burners, but they, too, work in less obvious ways. Aerobic workouts, such as brisk walking, running, swimming, and cycling, are the types of exercise that strengthen your heart and lungs and affect your cholesterol and other blood lipids most significantly. Like strengthening workouts, aerobic exercise impacts your metabolism positively. I'll talk more about each type of exercise and its benefits as we go on.

Life Spiraling Upward
Angela's Story

I was turning 40 and I was in a bad relationship—although I didn't even realize how bad it was till later. I had been an outgoing social person, but my controlling boyfriend had isolated me from my friends and family.

My weight crept up from 135 to 165. My self-confidence was shot, my self-esteem and self-worth were at an all-time low. Something had to change, but instead of recognizing that my relationship was the source of my misery, I thought I had to fix myself. I was searching for something to grab on to to drag me out of this bad place in my life, and I decided that it had to be something bigger than I could have ever imagined. So I picked the hardest thing I could think of: without ever having run a mile in my life, I decided to train for a marathon.

I hired a coach. I was reaching out for guidance, for support, for direction, but I was also reaching out for acceptance, strength, and a way to find myself. We ran four miles the first training session. I couldn't believe it; I didn't think that I could have run even a single mile. It felt great. I had just pushed the walls of the box that I had put myself in. What other walls needed to be broken down? What other walls had I put up?

I learned that during training you face a number of things: pain, self-doubt, your ego, your fears, your insecurities. But I also learned that the voice that says to you "I can't, I won't" slowly turns into "I can, I will." I am not sure who said this, but I use it all the time in my life and in my training. "Whether you think that you can—or think that you can't—you are right."

As my training progressed, my knees started to give me problems. My coach suggested that I try cross training on a bike to give my knees a break, and I took to it like a fish to water. I still run, but cycling became and still is my main activity.

It has been three years since I made the decision to train for a marathon. I haven't done a marathon (yet!), but I have ridden two 100-mile bike races and, in one of them, placed in the top 20 in my age group and in the top 100 women out of 6,000 people who entered the race. And I am still running. I have done one 5K, two 10Ks, and one biathlon, and two summers ago I rode the last half of the Tour de France (amateurs are allowed to ride part of the course early in the morning, before the professional cyclists catch up).

While I was out finding happiness on my bike, my life at home continued to spiral downward. My boyfriend, with whom

I had lived with for nine years, resented the time I spent running and cycling. He hated that I would come home from a workout and feel tired. "Most people manage to get a workout in thirty minutes. Why can't you?" he'd ask. At one point he gave me a bike, but he didn't want me to ride it! I'd sneak around and lie in order to work out and not tell him how far I was running or riding. I used to eat late to be with him and eat certain foods just to please him. He would buy food that I would ask him not to buy and even put doughnuts in my car and candy in my coat pockets. Knowing that I was training and trying to lose weight, he would make pasta every night for dinner and get angry if I didn't eat what he had made. He'd say, "You don't appreciate me, you're an ingrate!" I used to scrape the food off the plate and give it to the dogs when he wasn't looking.

One day, I realized that I wanted to be myself again. What I had long thought was love and attention from my boyfriend were really just his attempts to control me. He had an affair while I was in France riding the Tour. He said that it was my fault for leaving him alone for two weeks while I was selfishly off cycling. The hardest thing I could think of doing—riding the Tour de France—had now led me to the hardest thing in my life, the breakup of a bad relationship.

I don't think I would have had the strength to get through my breakup if I hadn't been training. Achieving all those things on the bike gave me clarity, strength, and self-esteem. And it introduced me to an entirely new set of people. I found happiness, friendship, love, and acceptance from people other than my boyfriend.

Once I had moved out, it seemed as if doors opened up for me, and the possibilities now seem endless. So many things about my life have changed. I now work for a company that I love, and after just eighteen months I've been promoted. I have taken back control of my life, and that includes what I eat. I still enjoy what I eat and eating out with family and friends, but I found that I needed a different combination of foods to help me achieve my goals. When a food tempts me, I say to myself, "Sure, I can eat this, but do I want to run faster and cycle farther?" If I answer yes, then I don't eat it. I eat small amounts all day long, and I have much more energy. I recently went to see a nutritionist and have visited a medical doctor who runs a longevity center. I'm trying to get information that will get me on the path to making the next forty years of my life the best of my life. My goal is to be 43, look 33, and feel 23!

I am now 130 pounds, and I'm surrounded by people who are supportive and who are living, training, and eating the same way I am—with focus, goals, positive lifestyles, and determination. I am also more direct and honest with myself and with my family now. I do what I need to do instead of doing what would please everyone else. I've learned to say no. I have inner strength and a core confidence; when you accomplish things like riding a hundred miles, it gives you the strength and the confidence to do other things. I have now been rock climbing and surfing. I've gained the mental and physical strength to do it all.

Yes, it is hard to eat the right things, not to overeat, to go to bed early to get up early and train. But I find that your achievements, goals, plans, and passions are delivered when you put in the work. You pay a price to make things better, but you also pay a price to stay where you are, to settle, to *not* do.

These days, instead of spiraling downward, I'm spiraling up. I have big goals. Maybe I can win that hundred-mile race one day. When you make the choice, when you make a decision, no matter how big or how small, you can shake off the things that are holding you back, and the sky's the limit. I made the choice to run, to ride, to compete, to train, to eat right, and to lose weight, to get away from someone destructive and controlling. I recommend that anyone contemplating change turn your thoughts into actions. Start right now.

Beyond Calorie Burning: How Else Exercise Contributes to Weight Loss and Good Health

My guess is that you already know that regular exercise can improve your cholesterol profile, especially by raising HDL—"good" cholesterol—levels, lower your blood pressure, and put you at a lower risk for heart disease, diabetes, and cancer, as well as other illnesses. You can experience many of the benefits of exercise without shedding pounds, but one of the main reasons exercise improves health is that it causes fat loss. Next to quitting smoking, getting your weight under control is the number one way to improve your physical well-being.

Weight loss occurs when the number of calories you burn is greater than the number of calories you take in. Exercise, obviously, helps increase the first half of that equation. Exercise more, burn more, lose more. But physical activity also affects your metabolism, the rate at which you burn calories, not just while you're working out but long after you've put away your sneakers.

Exercise boosts the metabolism in different ways. One way it does so is by increasing your muscle mass. Because muscle is a "calorie-hungry" tissue (it requires many times more calories than fat tissue to maintain), the more muscle you have, the more calories you'll burn even when you're just sitting around or sleeping. Another way exercise peps up your calorie burning is by providing a postworkout rise in metabolism. Cardio workouts, especially vigorous ones, can increase the rate at which you burn calories for up to ten hours after exercise. Strength training may do even more; one study found that it boosted metabolism for sixteen hours after a workout.

There's also another reason I think that exercise has a profound effect on the number of calories you burn: it's energizing. If you're new to exercise, you might find you're more tired than usual when you first begin working out, but eventually exercise is likely to make you feel stimulated and refreshed. And while having more energy won't necessarily increase the *rate* at which you burn calories, it may still increase the *number* you burn. Here's why: When you're energized, you'll have more stamina to perform the dozens of little extra calorie-burning moves you can do throughout the day. Things like getting up and going to talk to a colleague down the hall instead of sending an e-mail; taking the stairs instead of the elevator (both up and down); walking to the store instead of driving; rising from the couch to see why your kids are calling you instead of shouting to them from your comfortable perch. These are small things, but they all add up—and significantly. When scientists look at why some people burn more calories than others, they find that the high calorie burners are fidgeters. They're always moving in one way or another.

Keeping your metabolic fires burning is particularly important as you get older. Indeed, you may have already noticed that you have gained weight with each decade even if you haven't changed anything about the way you eat or the amount of activity you do. That's because a combination of changing hormones and diminishing muscle mass causes most people's metabolism to slow down by 2 to 10 percent per decade. And this doesn't just happen when you hit age 60; it begins in your twenties.

So, as you can see, the calorie-burning, metabolism-raising perks you get from exercise are not only essential to weight loss, they're critical in the ongoing fight we all wage against age-related weight gain. Consider, too, that both muscles and bones deteriorate with age if you don't do something to stop this process. Retaining muscle is vital because it will help you continue to be an active, vibrant person, as will preventing bone loss. The bones also tend to weaken as we get older, increasing the risk of fractures (women, because of the loss of estrogen after menopause, are particularly at risk). But weight-bearing exercise, especially strength training, can help bone to rebuild itself. There's absolutely no reason for us to become weak and feeble as we get older.

I also want to give you another reason to stick with exercise, not just for the duration of this 12-week program but for life: exercise has substantial psychological benefits. There are reams of studies showing that it lessens depression, stress, anxiety, tension, and anger. Some research has even shown that it works just as well as—and in some cases even better than—psychotherapy. If you're dealing with emotional issues, there's no substitute for doing the kind of soul-searching that I recommend in chapter 1. However, working out can assist you in working out your life problems. Many people (and I am one of them) swear to the fact that exercise helps them think more clearly and that they can even find solutions to problems while putting in time at the gym. The psychological benefits of exercise can't be overstated: it makes you feel good—and feel good about yourself.

Hooked on Exercise
Matt's Story

About a year and a half ago, I looked in the mirror and didn't like what I saw. My weight had risen to more than 200 pounds. I had high blood pressure and high cholesterol, which was particularly dispiriting since I have a family history of heart problems. So, at the age of 60, I made the decision to improve my physical, mental, and spiritual well-being. And I made it a Must, which is different from a Want.

I started slowly. I cut back on junk food and started drinking large amounts of water. I began walking one and a half miles every other day. After a while, I added in some push-ups, jumping jacks, and some moderate weight training, though I had no clue what I was doing. Still, after six months I began to clearly see some results. I looked better at 60 than I did at 30! I had the bug. And not just the "bug" in the sense that I was hooked, but the BUG: Begin Understanding Goals.

Some people close to me asked what I was doing all the exercise for. Others worried that working out was going to give me a heart attack. But you have to understand when someone tells me I can't do something, it makes me want to do it all that much more. So when I heard people's doubts, getting healthy became not only something to do for myself, it became a personal challenge.

Just to be on the safe side, I went to see my family doctor.

Much to my surprise and encouragement, this limited amount of exercise and weight training caused my cholesterol to drop from 298 to 154, my blood pressure from 140/95 to 117/63, and my weight from over 200 to 177 pounds. I could now see muscle where fat used to be. My doctor, instead of warning me not to tax my heart, encouraged me to continue the routines.

My next step was to find a fitness trainer. Twice a week for an hour and a half, Rich and I work on cardio and strength training, but his encouragement and coaching are what's most helpful. I am achieving the endurance, tone, and strength development of people half my age. After the workouts, I'm exhausted, but I walk out of the facility feeling as I can take on the world—at age 60! Every day (rain, shine, snow, heat) begins with a four-mile walk/jog.

Along with all this has come a dramatic change in the way I eat. I never used to eat anything before three o'clock; then I'd get hungry and have a Snickers bar in the late afternoon and maybe some fast food around five. Now I eat breakfast every day, oatmeal with skim milk. I eat balanced meals, lots of fruits and vegetables, a sandwich with chicken or turkey instead of the hoagies I used to eat. I haven't been to a fast-food restaurant in ages. I still eat pizza occasionally, and have a beer or wine once in a while. Ice cream and desserts? Almost never.

Life changes, not just physical changes, have clearly occurred since that time I first looked in the mirror and didn't like what I saw. My self-confidence, both at work and in social circles, has increased significantly. Stress is almost a thing of the past, and when it does occur, it's manageable. I'm gearing up to run my first 8K—at age 60!—and I'm determined to place in the top four of my age class.

Throughout all this, I have also experienced profound spiritual growth. I see life as a gift from a higher power, and I think it's important to appreciate the gift and take care of it. The BUG is alive, well, and nourished, and so am I.

Consistency Is Key

It's sometimes said that it doesn't matter what kind of or how much exercise you do as long as you're consistent about it. I don't quite agree; if you're looking to make your body over, it *does* matter what and how much of it you do. But I do agree that consistency is key. You really need to exercise six days a week, every week. Exercise must be as integral to your life as taking a daily shower and brushing your teeth.

If you are a longtime regular exerciser, you've probably already learned that you need to build it into your life and stay with it. If you have never exercised or have started and stopped a hundred times, you need to commit to maintaining a consistent program. Of course, there will be occasions when you miss a workout or even two. However, it's essential that you not let it turn into three, four, or even more days. It's not uncommon for people who have missed their workouts to feel angry at themselves for slipping up, then to let that anger boil up into defeat. "Why keep at it when I obviously can't stick to a schedule?" they ask themselves. That's the absolute wrong attitude. So you missed a few workouts? You're not going to lose a lot of fitness in a few days, but you will if you let it stretch into a week or more. That will take you back to square one, and it'll be all that much harder when you begin again.

Don't let missed workouts make you feel as if you might as well eat whatever you want because you have to start over anyway. Be 99 percent consistent, deal with the little inconsistencies, and get back on track. Pledge to yourself right now that when you embark upon this program, you're in it for every day of those 12 weeks. Stay with it, and it will be all that much easier to transition into being active for the rest of your life.

Where to Begin: At What Level Are You?

The effects of this 12-week program will be greatly enhanced if you choose the plan that's right for your level of fitness. You don't want the amount of exercise to be too easy or too hard, you want to get it just right. The beauty of it, especially for beginners and intermediate exercisers, is that once you finish the 12 weeks you will officially be at the next level; beginners will be intermediates; intermediates will be advanced; advanced, well, you'll be more advanced! Beginners and intermediates, your next step might even be to go through the 12 weeks again, the second time at the next level. As I said, though, be sure to slot yourself into the right category at the outset. Here are some guidelines to help you.

Beginners, you most likely know who you are. You may not ever have participated in an exercise program beyond having to take PE class in school. Or if you have, it might have been so long ago that you're pretty much back at square one. Beginners get out of breath at the slightest exertion, and your lack of strength keeps you from doing even some minor tasks, such as moving a chair or lifting a child. But say you can move a chair and lift children; does that disqualify you from beginner status? Not necessarily. Many times people develop some strength out of necessity. If the work you do in your garden requires that you frequently cart dirt around, your arms and shoulders may have gotten strong. But what about the rest of you? Your goal here is to acquire a *total* body makeover, which means you're going to need to hit every part of your body, so evaluate your *total* fitness when deciding if you're a beginner or not.

If you're an **intermediate** exerciser, you probably already have a fitness routine going. You may routinely work out at least three times a week and have done some weight training, too. But there's a good chance you've reached a plateau. The exercise you're doing isn't helping you change your body, and it's become a little too easy.

People at an **advanced** level are already very committed to working out. If you already strength train three or four times a week, do at least 45 minutes of aerobic exercise per exercise session, and perhaps even take part in more than one type of cardio exercise, this is the category to which you belong. Like the intermediate exerciser, you may have hit a wall and are not seeing the changes you want. Or perhaps you just want the challenge of kicking your exercise program up to the next level or to add some variety to the exercises you currently perform. In either case, think of this 12-week program as boot camp: an intense training period during which you can get into your best shape ever.

Increasing the Challenge: What You Need to Know About Progressing

You don't really have to think too much about how to progress during the next 12 weeks, because your goals for each week are laid out for you. Just turn to the page of the week you're on, and you'll see what you're expected to accomplish during those seven days. Still, I'd like to give you an idea of what you're going to be doing and what the progression will be like. You can read about the specific exercises in the pages that follow, but here's an at-a-glance guide to your program. (Note: All the references to intensity and sets will be clearer once you have read the next section "Fitness Basics.")

BEGINNERS
WEEKS 1–12

TYPE OF EXERCISE	HOW MUCH TO START	HOW OFTEN	RATE OF PROGRESS
Functional fitness exercises	Exercises 1–11, 1–2 sets (or 2–3 stretches)	6 times a week	At 7 weeks, up the number of sets
Strength-training exercises	Exercises 1–8, 1–2 sets	3 times a week	At 7 weeks, up the number of sets; add exercises 9–10
Aerobic workouts	15 minutes or as much as you can do	5 days a week at a 7–8 intensity	Increase by 2 minutes each week
Double aerobic workouts	30 minutes or as much as you can do	1 day a week at a 6–7 intensity	Continue to double your regular aerobic workout time

INTERMEDIATE
WEEKS 1–12

TYPE OF EXERCISE	HOW MUCH TO START	HOW OFTEN	RATE OF PROGRESS
Functional fitness exercises	Exercises 1–11, 3 sets (or 3 stretches)	6 times a week	No change
Strength-training exercises	Exercises 1–13, 3 sets	3 times a week	At 7 weeks, increase to every other day; add exercises 14–15
Aerobic workouts	30 minutes	5 days a week at a 7–8 intensity	Increase by 2 minutes each week
Double aerobic workouts	60 minutes	1 day a week at a 6–7 intensity	Continue to double your regular aerobic workout time

ADVANCED
WEEKS 1–12

TYPE OF EXERCISE	HOW MUCH TO START	HOW OFTEN	RATE OF PROGRESS
Functional fitness exercises	Exercises 1–15, 3 sets (or 3 stretches)	6 times a week	No change
Strength-training exercises	Exercises 1–15, 3 sets	Every other day	At week 7, add exercises 16–19
Aerobic workouts	45 minutes	5 days a week at a 7–8 intensity	Increase by 2 minutes each week
Double aerobic workouts	90 minutes	1 day a week at a 6–7 intensity	Continue to double your regular aerobic workout time

As you make your way through the program, it's important to check in with yourself before you automatically take on the next week's challenges. No matter what's on the schedule, if you're not ready to go from, say, week six to week seven, by all means stay where you are. That goes for everyone, whether you're a beginner or an advanced exerciser. I don't want working out to become too easy for you, or you won't get the changes you're hoping for. But neither do I want you to push yourself to an unhealthy limit. Each week you'll need to judge how you feel and ask yourself these questions before you move on:

- Was I *solidly* meeting the exercise prescription for this week, or was it a struggle?
- Did the exercise make me feel unusually tired?
- Did I have any trouble getting my heart rate to come down after the aerobic workouts?
- Am I having trouble sleeping?

There is nothing wrong with hanging back a week or even more if you need to. What's most important is that you completely master each step along the way. If you try to build before you're ready, you will likely feel awful and be tempted to give it all up. Worse, you may injure yourself. I think the progression I have charted for you will be doable, but in the end, you must be the judge and move on when only you feel you're ready.

From Fitness Dabbler to Fitness Dynamo
Elizabeth's Story

I'm probably not your typical weight loss success story, because when I accepted Bob's challenge to make some life changes a few years ago, I was only about ten pounds overweight. I was already doing some exercising; the trouble was, I wasn't doing anything consistently. Sometimes I would eat healthfully, sometimes I wouldn't. Sometimes I would stick to a fitness regimen, sometimes I wouldn't. The other problem was that I was obsessed with my body image. I felt as though I never looked good enough. I drove my husband crazy: "Do I look fat in this?" "Is my butt too big?" It wasn't until I heard my six-year-old daughter say that she thought a certain skirt made her look too big that I woke up. I knew I had to get comfortable in my own skin. I took Bob's challenge and literally ran with it.

My goal was to make my body fit and strong through exercise. I was hoping that I could improve my sense of myself by doing something that I knew was healthy and, in the meantime, set a good example for my two daughters. I want my girls to be raised by someone they see as strong and healthy.

My biggest obstacle was the one so many people face: time. I didn't have enough of it. So I tried to be creative. When I dropped my youngest daughter off at preschool, I made sure I was dressed and ready to hit the gym right afterward. The time I was taking for the workouts definitely took time away from my other responsibilities at home, but I realized I had to carve out the hour because it made me happy—and if I wasn't happy, no one at home was going to be happy either. I began by lifting weights two days at the gym and two days at home.

Next came cardio. I got up at 5 A.M. so that I could run on our brand-new treadmill. I was motivated to get up not only because I wanted to see changes in my body and become more heart healthy, but because we had spent money out of the family budget on it. I'm way too frugal to waste it!

The more physical I became, the more I started thinking about how I was fueling both my body and the bodies of my husband and kids. I stopped buying convenience foods like chips and instead bought vegetables that the kids could dip in ranch dressing. I also started cooking a lot of vegetarian meals and learning more about legumes and tofu.

Eventually, I extended healthy changes to the time I spent with my family and friends. Now instead of a dinner and movie, my husband and I will spend our precious time together doing active things like Rollerblading and canoeing. I've planned evenings with girlfriends that involve going to the gym. My girlfriends and I have even taken weekend biking trips together. I have started running races and have asked others to join me. My husband rode his bike along with me during one half marathon, and my eldest daughter and I participated in a Race for the Cure event. I convinced a friend who never thought of herself as a runner to train for a half marathon with me. (Turns out she's faster than me, and now I'm the one who has to work hard to keep up.)

Because of the exercise and my new eating habits, I've lost ten pounds, but who cares? More important, I've reached my goal of feeling better about myself. I'm far less obsessed with my body image, and just knowing that I'm strong and healthy—I can lift an 80-pound water softener bag!—has made me more confident.

I am very aware of how I am fueling my body and what effects it will have not only on the scale but on my workouts.

For example, in the past I might eat Cheetos with the kids, but now I realize that for me it's a choice. I can eat the Cheetos (and sometimes I do!) and enjoy them, or I can skip the Cheetos or reach for an apple as a better choice. I have also learned to avoid alcohol. I've never been a big drinker, though I do enjoy a great glass of wine with a meal. I can have the wine, but I realize it will affect the way I feel when I run for the next two days—it affects my speed, distance, and general sense of well-being.

One thing that has been the most fun for me in my pursuit of healthier living is all the connections I've made with other people. I have developed a group of girlfriends I can exercise with and also learn from. I value the time I have with my girlfriends, and when I can combine this with what else I value—exercise—it's a complete win-win!

I am also very fortunate to have a supportive husband who respects the time I spend taking care of myself. He recognizes the benefits to our family. He has also has learned to value his own time working out and playing hockey. He knows he doesn't have to feel guilty about taking time away to take care of himself too.

I feel as though I will continue to learn more as I go, but I already feel that I'm not doomed to be a grandparent who sits on the sidelines, but rather one who goes on the monkey bars with the kids. I believe I'm like a lot of other people out there, but the difference is that I wasn't afraid to try to change. I didn't dip my toe in the water, I jumped in and went swimming. Turns out the water is fine!

Fitness Basics

The next 12 weeks are going to be incredibly challenging, yet also invigorating. You are standing on the threshold of a whole new life, and even the fact that you've gotten this far—that is, you've asked yourself the hard questions and made the commitment to change—should help build your confidence. As you go forward, think about the success stories you've been reading and use them to inspire you to stay on track. Once you prove to yourself you can push through the temptations and tough spots, you can be your own inspiration. You'll be proud of your accomplishments—and rightfully so!

So here's what you're in for during the next 12 weeks; all the elements of the program are described in detail. Familiarize yourself with all the exercises and read through the information about how they'll help you achieve a total body makeover. The more you understand about the way the exercises work, the more what you're doing will make sense to you.

Whether your goal is to lose 100 pounds or to drop just a stubborn 10, whether you just want to make exercise more of a priority in your life and eat a more nutritious diet or you are already health-conscious and just want to get superfit, this program is going to get you there. You may not reach your ultimate goal in 12 if you have a lot of weight to lose, but you'll be on the road to success. The work you'll be doing will be hard, but the rewards will be substantial. Stick with each component of the program, and you'll be on the path to changing your body for good.

Functional Exercise

"Functional fitness" is a daunting phrase that actually refers to something very basic: how well you're able to do all the physical tasks you need to do each day. Being functionally fit means being able to carry bags of groceries without strain, to bend down and pick up laundry off the floor without pulling a muscle, to lift a child without injuring your back, to walk around a city while sightseeing without becoming so sore that you ruin the rest of your vacation. After all, what good is being able to lift an impressive amount of weight in the gym if you can't reach for something in the back of your closet without throwing out your back?

A lot of what contributes to functional fitness is flexibility. Simply staying active—moving—loosens up the body and improves flexibility, but working some stretching exercises into your routine will help you take it a step further. Even if you already stretch regularly, take a look at my functional stretches. They are designed to elongate the biggest muscles of the body and, together, provide a good allover body tune-up.

If you have read any of my other books, the following exercises might look familiar. While I've tried tons of other exercises, I still think these give you the most bang for the buck. They're simple yet effective.

Stretching

Flexibility refers to the ability of the muscles and joints to give and thus allow us to move more freely. Stretching, because it helps the muscles release, improves flexibility. Whether or not it has other benefits (such as improving athletic performance, preventing postexercise soreness, and reducing the risk of injury) has been extensively studied and hotly debated by researchers, but with little consensus. At the very least, I think stretching does help to prevent the stiffness that can make going about your day-to-day life uncomfortable. Plus, it really feels good, and gives you a few moments to take a time out after exercise, to renew yourself and reflect on the session you've just completed.

I say "after exercise" because contrary to what many people believe, that's the best time to stretch. It's very easy to injure muscles that are cold. Just think how resistant to stretch cold taffy is and how easily it can be elongated when warm. Your muscles are the same way, so save your stretching routine until after you've done your cardio or strength-training workout. If you have the time, gentle stretching before a workout can also be helpful. But if you're going to do so, warm up your body first by walking or getting onto a cardiovascular machine, such as a treadmill, stationary bike, or elliptical trainer, until you break a sweat, about five to ten minutes.

It's also a good idea to do some stretches throughout the day. You might, for instance, simply bend over, place your hands on a wall, and give your back a stretch after sitting a long time at your desk. Or stand in a doorway, spread your arms, place your hands on the doorjamb and lean forward to stretch your shoulders and chest. You don't need to warm up for these stretches; they should be done gently, the goal being just to help your body loosen up after remaining in one position for a long time. Think of the natural inclination you have to stretch when you wake up in the morning, and carry that with you throughout your day.

There's actually some technique involved in stretching, though it seems very simple. Years ago, bouncing up and down in a stretch—called ballistic stretching—was considered optimal, until it was found it could lead to injury. Most people now use the static technique, the kind that requires holding the stretch for about 20 to 30 seconds or even longer. I prefer a different type of stretching. Instead of holding the stretch for a long time, I hold it for five seconds, relax for two seconds, then stretch again for five seconds. I repeat this pattern for about two minutes for each stretch. Although static stretching works very well, I think this hold-and-release method works a little better. When you stretch, your muscles, in an effort to protect themselves, actually resist the tension, allowing you to stretch only so far. When you stretch, then quickly relax, the resistance relaxes too, allowing you to go deeper into the move during the next four-second stretch. If you try the static method, then compare it to the hold-and-release method, I think you'll see the difference in how much further the latter technique helps you stretch.

Stabilizing Exercises

The functional exercises you'll be doing each week also include some abdominal, back, shoulder, and lower leg exercises. These exercises are often considered strength-training moves, as they do act to strengthen. However, I like to think of them as functional exercises because (a) having a strong core is so central to every aspect of your physical being, and (b) having strong shoulders and lower legs will help you avoid injury when you begin doing the more taxing exercises.

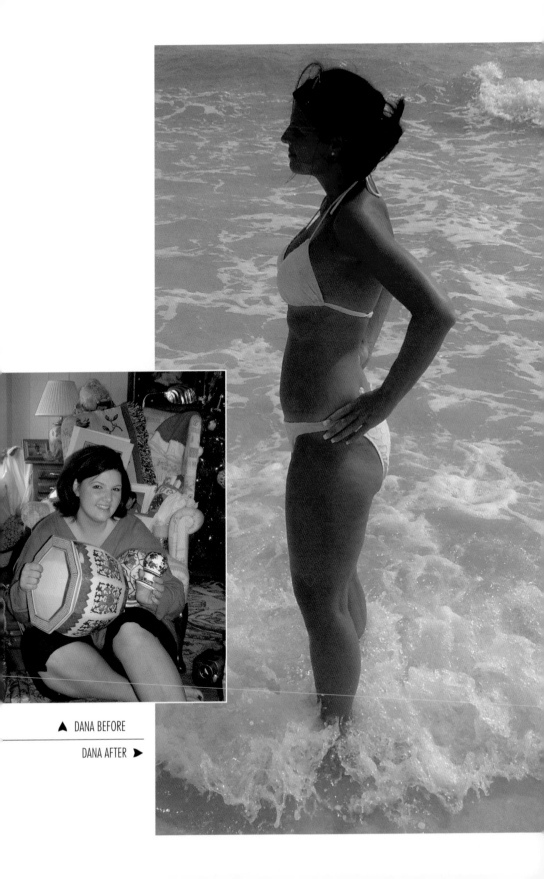

▲ DANA BEFORE

DANA AFTER ▶

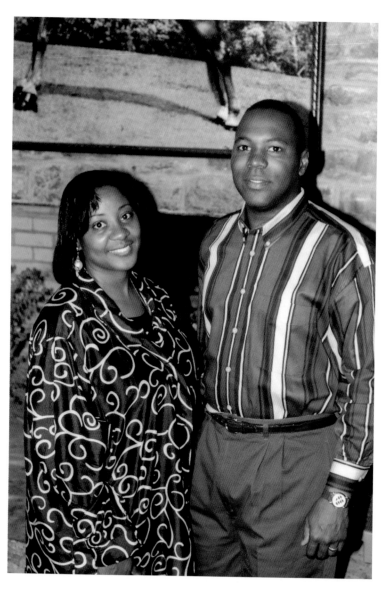

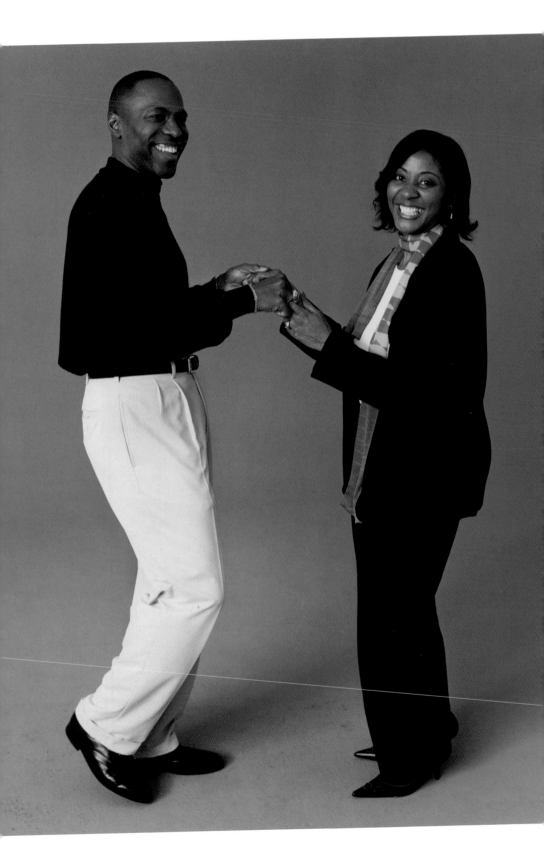

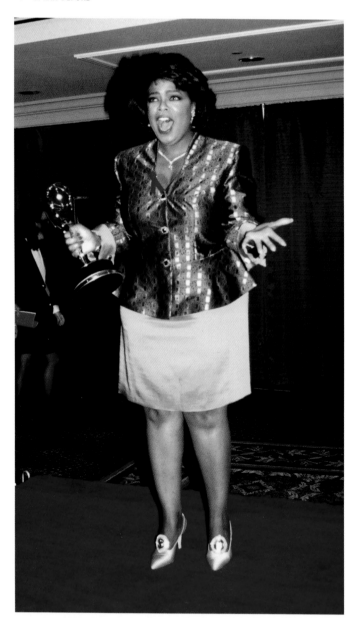

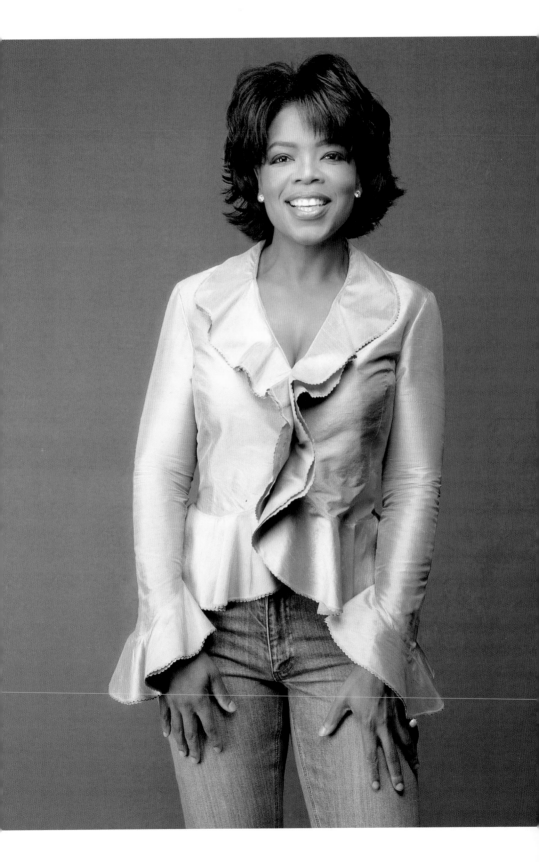

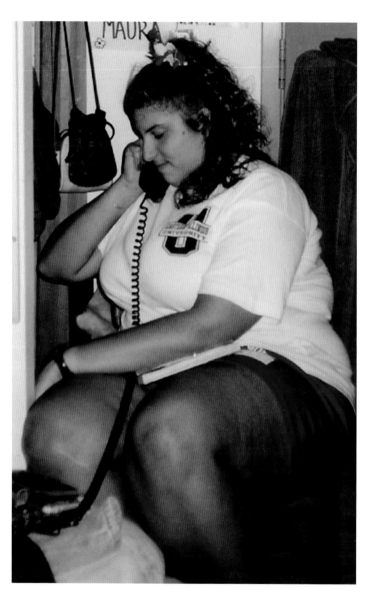

▲ RENÉE BEFORE

RENÉE AFTER ▶

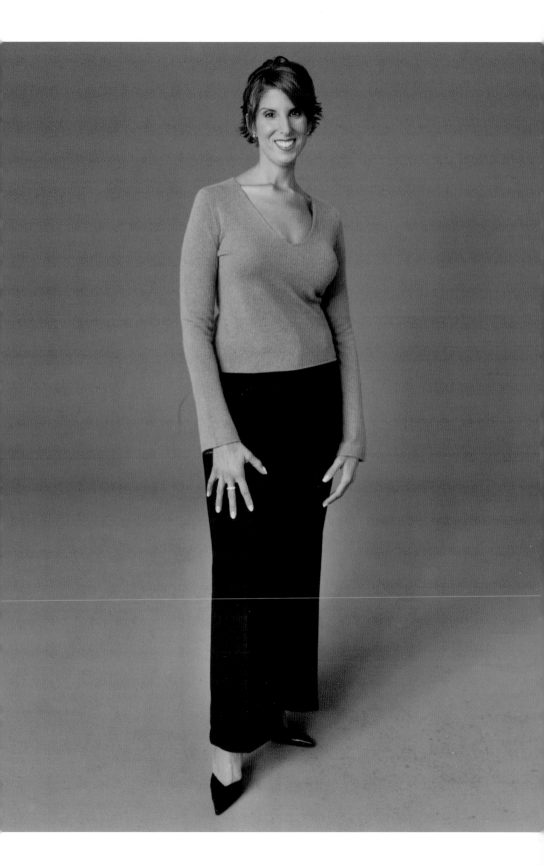

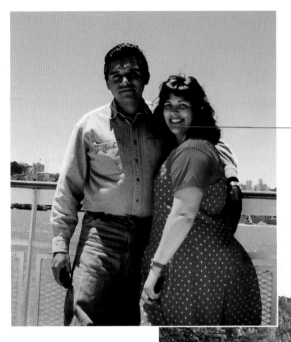

▲ TAWNI BEFORE

TAWNI AFTER ▶

Having strong abs and a strong back, in particular, helps protect your spine from daily wear and tear. Having a strong midsection will also enhance your ability to do every other fitness activity, from walking to weight training. Few people realize it, but just about every move we make engages or initiates from the core of the body. Perhaps that's why the abdominal muscles are often neglected. Unless they're going for the classic "six-pack," most people give the abs a pass.

While we're on the subject, there are a few misconceptions about abdominal exercises that I'd like to clear up. The first is that you need to do hundreds upon hundreds of sit-ups to see any results. Despite the fact that sit-up overkill seems to be a point of pride for some people, it's somewhat of a waste of time. A good, effective range of abdominal exercises will do the job with far fewer repetitions—generally 15 reps each exercise and anywhere from one to three sets depending on your level of fitness. If you're doing a whole lot more than that, your form will probably suffer and you won't get the benefits of the exercises. A better strategy than racking up the repetitions is to increase the difficulty, which you can do by adding on sets, using an incline bench, or using a weight.

Another fallacy about abdominal exercises is that they will give you a flat abdomen. Unfortunately, working your middle won't whittle it down—losing fat is the only way to do that, and burning more calories than you consume is the only way to lose fat. But abdominal exercises *will* strengthen your abdomen, improving your posture and the way you carry yourself. This will enhance the way you look, no doubt about it. Further, as you begin to lose fat and your abdominal muscles come into view, you will have a firmer, better-looking middle. Just don't count on crunches alone to make the fat disappear.

Like abdominal exercises, the lower leg exercises you'll be doing are also important for preventing injury, in particular shin splints, an inflammatory condition that can be painful and debilitating. Walking, jogging, climbing stairs—anything that involves pounding your lower legs against the ground—can give you shin splints. Preventive strengtheners, stretches, and a proper warmup will help you avoid them.

The Exercises

Equipment needs: A floor mat and, as you progress, dumbbells. Advanced exercisers will also need an incline board.

Stretches

Throughout each stretch, breathe deeply but naturally.

1. Hamstring Stretch

The setup: While standing, put your hands on your hips and place one foot on a chair with the toes of that foot pointing toward the ceiling. Keep both legs straight, with your knees locked but not hyperextended.

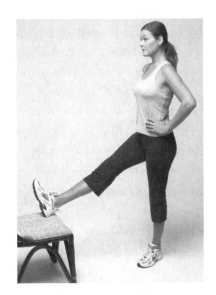

Starting position

The move: Gradually bend forward until you feel a gentle tension in the back of the thigh (your hamstring) of the elevated leg. Hold for 5 seconds; relax for 5 seconds; repeat two more times. Switch legs.

Tip: As you bend forward, keep your back straight.

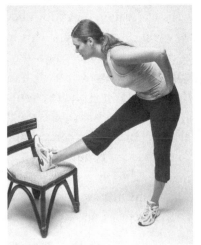

Active phase

2. Quadriceps Stretch

The setup: With one hand, hold on to a chair for support. Use your other hand to grab the ankle of the same-side leg as you bend it and bring your heel toward your buttocks.

The move: Keeping the knee of your opposite leg slightly bent and your knees parallel, gently bring your heel in closer toward your buttocks until you feel moderate tension in the front of your thigh. Hold for 5 seconds; relax for 5 seconds; repeat two times. Switch sides.

Tip: Be careful not to overarch your back as you go.

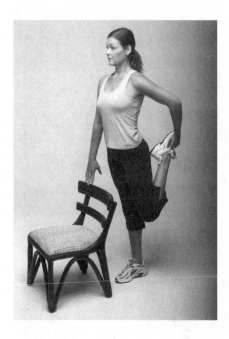

3. Upper Calf Stretch

The setup: With one hand, hold on to a chair for support. Place your other hand on your hip and slide one leg straight out behind you about two feet, keeping the heel on the ground.

The move: Bend your front leg slightly while keeping your knee directly over the corresponding foot (don't let your knee extend past your foot). You should feel gentle tension in the upper calf of your back leg. If you don't, bring your front leg farther forward. Hold for 5 seconds; relax for 5 seconds; repeat two times. Switch sides.

Tip: Keep your feet firmly planted on the ground; avoid arching your back.

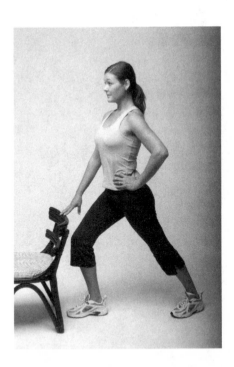

4. Lower Calf Stretch

The setup: With one hand, hold on to a chair for support. Place your other hand on your hip and slide one leg straight out behind you about two feet, keeping the heel on the ground.

The move: Bend both knees and slowly bring your hips toward the floor, keeping both heels on the ground. You should feel a gentle tension in the lower calf of your back leg. Hold for 5 seconds; relax for 5 seconds; repeat two times. Switch sides.

Tip: Keep your feet firmly planted on the ground; avoid arching your back.

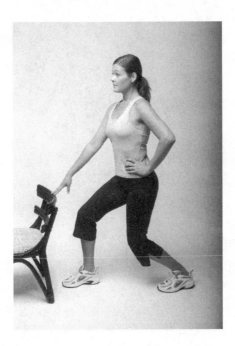

5. Middle and Lower Back Stretch

The setup: Sit on a chair with your knees slightly more than hip width apart and stretch your arms out in front of you.

The move: Gradually bend forward, keeping your arms stretched out and between your knees. Reach down toward the floor until you feel a gentle tension in your upper and/or middle back. Hold for 5 seconds; relax for 5 seconds; repeat two times.

Tip: To increase the stretch, draw in your abdominal muscles and let your upper back move even further forward.

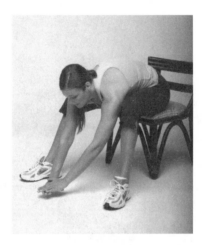

Stabilizing Exercises

Although I consider these functional exercises, they primarily help you gain strength, so a lot of the rules for strength training apply here as well. See page 119–120 in the strength-training section for information on repetitions and sets.

Abdominal Exercises

During these exercises, exhale on your way up and inhale as you return to the starting position.

6. Basic Crunches

The setup: Lie faceup on the floor with your knees bent and your heels 12 to 15 inches from your buttocks. Clasp your hands lightly behind your neck.

The move: Using your abdominal muscles to power you, raise your torso to a 30- to 45-degree angle. Your chin should point straight up toward the ceiling. Pause for a second before returning to the starting position. Repeat until the entire set is complete

Tips: Don't let your neck roll as you rise up, and keep your shoulders square throughout the entire exercise. Once your neck is strengthened (typically within a month of beginning to perform this exercise), try resting your hands lightly on your collarbone instead of clasping them behind your neck.

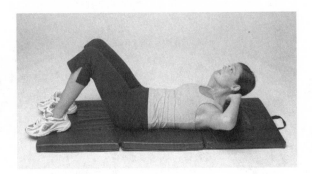

With neck supported

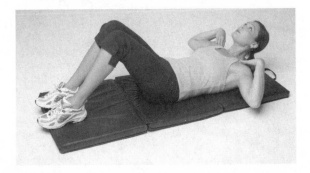

With neck unsupported

7. Twisting Trunk Curl Crunches

The setup: Lie faceup on the floor with your knees bent and your heels 12 to 15 inches from your butt. Place your left ankle on your right knee and clasp your hands lightly behind your neck.

The move: Using your abdominal muscles to power you, raise your right shoulder toward your left knee. Your shoulder should lift only 8 to 12 inches off the floor. Pause for a second at the top, then return to the floor. Repeat until the entire set is complete. Switch sides.

Tip: Use the arm on the floor as a pivot point as you rise up toward your knees.

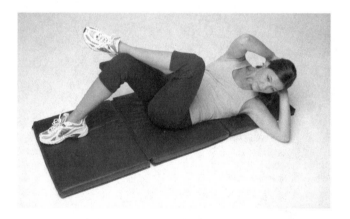

8. Upper Abdomen Crunches

The setup: Lie faceup on the floor. Raise your legs and bend them at a 90-degree angle. It's a good idea to support your legs on a chair or exercise ball or to place your feet on a wall until you are strong enough to hold them at a 90-degree angle on your own. Clasp your hands lightly behind your neck.

The move: Using your abdominal muscles to power you, raise your torso off the floor to a 30- to 45-degree angle. Your chin should point straight up toward the ceiling. Pause for a second before returning to the starting position. Repeat until the entire set is complete.

Tip: Don't let your neck roll as you rise up, and keep your shoulders square throughout the entire exercise. Once your neck is strengthened (typically within a month of beginning to perform this exercise), try resting your hands lightly on your collarbone instead of clasping them behind your neck.

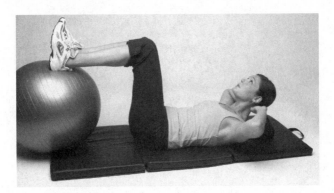

With neck and legs supported

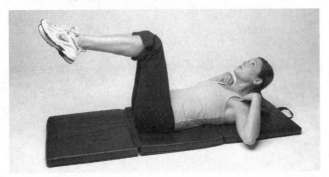

With neck and legs unsupported

Back and Shoulder Exercises

9. Arm and Leg Raise

The setup: Lie facedown on the floor with your head supported by a folded towel and your arms extended over your head.

The move: Contract your abdominal muscles and the muscles of your lower back. Raise your right arm and your left leg simultaneously, keeping your shoulders and pelvis pressed against the floor. Lift only until you feel a gentle tension in your lower back muscles. Pause for a second before returning to the starting position. Exhale on your way up, and inhale on your way back down. Repeat until the entire set is complete; switch sides and repeat.

Tip: Be sure to keep your nonworking leg and your head down.

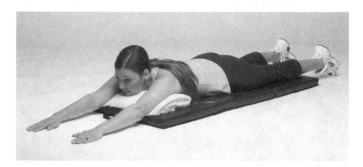

Starting position

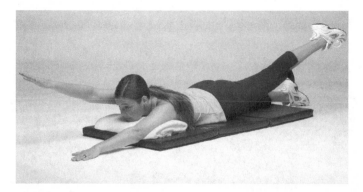

Active phase

10. Shrug Roll

The setup: Stand tall, with your feet slightly apart and your arms at your sides.

The move: Begin the exercise by bringing your shoulders up toward your ears as high as they will go. Pause for a second at the top of this motion, then roll your shoulders back while squeezing your shoulder blades together. Again pause for a second, then drop your shoulders back to the starting position. Breathe naturally throughout the exercise. Continue until the entire set is complete.

Tip: Keep your posture natural, neither ramrod straight or arched; add dumbbells to this exercise as you progress to increase the difficulty. (Beginners, add two- or three-pound dumbbells after about four weeks of starting this exercise.)

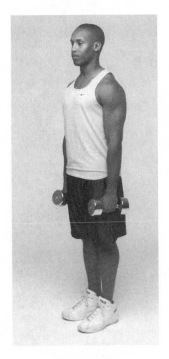 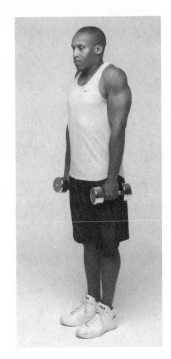

Starting position   *Active phase*

Lower Leg Exercises

11. Heel Raises

The setup: This exercise is best performed standing on a board approximately 2 inches by 6 inches by 36 inches or any slightly raised, stable surface. Stand tall, with your feet slightly apart and your knees straight but not hyperextended. Place the ball of each foot on the raised surface and your heels on the floor.

The move: Slowly raise your heels as high as possible and hold for a split second before slowly returning to the starting position. Continue until the entire set is complete.

Tip: Keep your posture natural, neither ramrod straight or arched; dumbbells will be added to this exercise as you progress to increase the difficulty. (Beginners, add three-pound dumbbells after about four weeks of starting this exercise.)

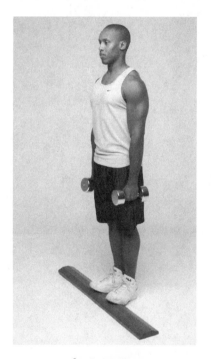

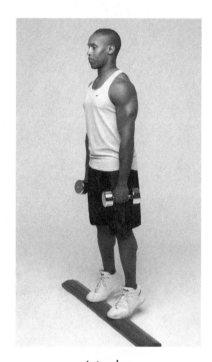

Starting position   *Active phase*

Advanced Only

12. Reverse Trunk Curl

The setup: Lie faceup on the floor with your legs straight up, perpendicular to the ground, your knees bent slightly. Keep your hands palm down at your sides. Your entire back and your shoulder blades should remain flat on the floor.

The move: Contract your abdominal muscles; then curl your pelvis up so that your feet go up toward the ceiling. Raise your hips only 3 to 5 inches off the floor. Pause for a second before returning to starting position. Repeat until the entire set is complete.

Tip: Be sure your legs and buttocks remain relaxed; the primary work should be done by your abdominal muscles. This one takes some practice; if you've never done it before, you may have to gradually build up to completing an entire set.

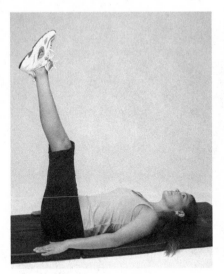
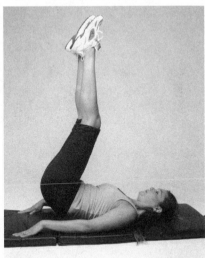

Starting position   *Active phase*

Advanced Only

13. Extended Arm Crunch

The setup: Lie faceup on the floor with your knees bent and your heels 12 to 15 inches from your buttocks. Place one hand behind your neck for support. Extend the other arm straight out so that it is between your knees.

The move: Contract your abdominal muscles and use them to raise your torso off the floor to a 30- to 45-degree angle. Your chin should go straight up toward the ceiling with no rolling of your neck. Pause for a second before returning to the starting position. Repeat until the entire set is complete.

Tip: As your neck is strengthened, you can extend both arms straight out.

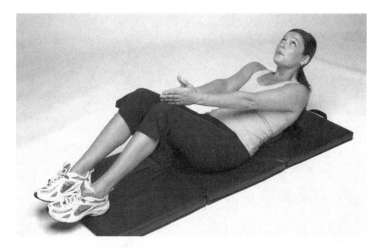

Active phase with neck unsupported

Advanced Only

14. Vertical Leg Crunch

The setup: Lie faceup on the floor with your legs straight up, perpendicular to the ground, your knees bent slightly. Place your palms lightly behind your neck.

The move: Contract your abdominal muscles and use them to raise your torso off the floor to a 30- to 45-degree angle. Your chin should go straight up toward the ceiling with no rolling of your neck. Pause for a second before returning to the starting position. Continue until the entire set is complete.

Tip: As your neck gets stronger, you can extend both arms straight out.

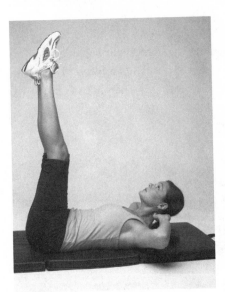 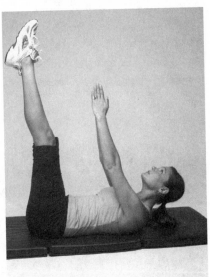

With neck supported   *With neck unsupported*

Advanced Only

15. Incline Sit-Up

The setup: Lie faceup on an incline board with your knees bent and your heels 12 to 15 inches from your buttocks, or hooked under the board's leg pads. Allow your hands to rest gently on your collarbone with your elbows out to the side. Your back should be flat against the pad of the board and your feet locked under the footholds.

The move: Using your abdominal muscles to power you, raise your torso to a 30- to 45-degree angle. Your chin should point straight up toward the ceiling. Pause for a second before returning to the starting position. Repeat until the entire set is complete. You should perform 15 to 50 repetitions in each set according to your ability.

Tip: Don't let your neck roll as you rise up, and keep your shoulders square throughout the entire exercise. Most incline boards have three or four settings. Do each set on a different setting, increasing the height as you go.

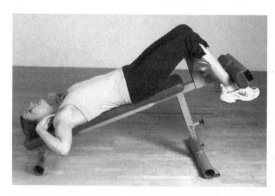

Starting position

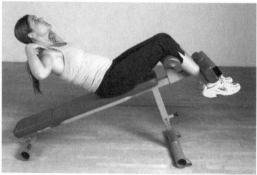

Active phase

YOGA AND PILATES
Workouts You Might Want to Try

If you have time, yoga and Pilates are great additions to this program, or you may want to take them up after the 12 weeks are through. Besides providing fitness benefits, both of these workouts emphasize concentration and focus and, in doing so, not only make you more aware of how you move and hold your body but also let you block out the rest of the world as you exercise. They are, in a sense, meditation in motion, and because they both improve flexibility and balance, they fit nicely into the functional fitness category.

I think of both yoga and Pilates as icing on the fitness cake. They're not substitutes for other functional fitness exercises, nor are they substitutes for strength training and cardiovascular exercise. Still, yoga and Pilates are both excellent adjuncts to a traditional fitness regime.

There are plenty of ways to get a yoga or Pilates program going: classes, videotapes or DVDs, audiotapes, books. Here's what you should know about each discipline to find the workout that's right for you.

Yoga

Despite its reputation, yoga is not about twisting your body into positions that seemingly defy anatomy; in fact, you don't even have to be particularly limber to do it. Instead, it's an activity that involves finding your body's limits, then trying to reach beyond them, using breathing and intense concentration to guide you.

Yoga is probably best known and loved for the poses that stretch the body, loosening up tight muscles and helping release tension in the bargain. But many poses also test and develop balance, while others rely more on strength. Moreover, there are many different styles of the physical practice of yoga (the word "yoga" also applies to practices of devotion and philosophy), so there's a good chance you'll find one that suits your own style.

When choosing a class or home workout, it's important to select instruction that matches your ability. In other words, don't go to a level three class if you've never taken yoga before—even if you are extremely fit you may find it very difficult and possibly end up injured. Also, keep in mind that because the practice of yoga is so varied it may take you awhile to find a style or a teacher you like. Don't give up after one or two different classes. You'll also need to consider how spiritual you want your practice to be. Some classes involve chanting and meditation; others are just straight physical exercise.

Pilates

This fitness regimen is based on a series of calisthenics-like moves performed on a mat or with the aid of various apparatus. The Pilates machines—the most famous is one called a "reformer"—sometimes look kind of like homemade contraptions but actually work quite well to help you move fluidly in the face of resistance. Pilates moves are very graceful and are done slowly in a controlled fashion, each move flowing easily into the next. At various points along the way, you're called on to contract, then elongate your muscles; the elongation is a little bit like ballet. Some exercises even call for keeping the feet in "Pilates stance," a modified version of a balletic turnout (heels together, toes pointing outward).

The primary goal of Pilates is to strengthen what Pilates teachers refer to as the "powerhouse," a wide belt around the body's middle that includes the muscles in the stomach, hips, lower back, and buttocks. In fact, every Pilates exercise engages the abdominal muscles, and, by helping you strengthen your core, the workout improves posture and balance, reducing the risk of backaches and other pain. People who practice the regimen like the way it lengthens their bodies and helps train them to keep their abdominal muscles taut at all times.

Aerobic Exercise

Aerobic or cardiovascular exercise (the terms are used interchangeably) is where serious calorie burning comes into play. But there's quite a bit more to it than that, and I think that the mechanics of aerobic exercise—any kind of rhythmic, continuous exercise that causes you to consume a large amount of oxygen for an extended period of time—should be a part of your basic health knowledge.

One of the benefits of regular aerobic exercise is endurance. "Aerobic" means "with oxygen," so it's not surprising that the demands you make on your body when you ask it to sustain an aerobic activity train your lungs to deliver oxygen and your heart to pump out greater amounts of blood to carry that oxygen to your working muscles. Your body also responds to this challenge by producing and storing something referred to as aerobic enzymes. These enzymes help you burn more fat, another reason why aerobic exercise has such a pronounced effect on your body fat. This effect, which is often overlooked, is a primary reason why people doing aerobic exercise establish a new metabolism and a leaner body.

Yet another benefit of aerobic training is that it enables your muscles to better use oxygen to perform work over extended periods of time. That translates into endurance, so with regular exercise you'll be able to perform without gasping madly for breath or tiring out after only a few minutes.

As the physiological changes in your body make it possible for you to exercise without huffing and puffing, they also improve your health. Aerobic exercise increases HDL (good) cholesterol and reduces blood pressure, increases insulin sensitivity (thereby reducing your risk of developing diabetes), and seems to provide some protection against cancer. By increasing circulation, it also helps your skin and hair stay healthy. And by causing the release of certain brain chemicals, it can even inhibit the stress hormones that might be surreptitiously taking a toll on your well-being.

Then, of course, there are the calorie-burning benefits of aerobic exercise. How many calories you burn during a session depends on how long and how vigorous the session is. The intensity of the exercise also influences the session's "afterburn"—the temporary boost in your metabolism postexercise. But there's also another, more permanent effect: when you get very fit, the rate at which you burn calories stays elevated permanently. You actually change your metabolism, which is the primary goal of this program.

Most people want to know the bottom line about aerobic exercise: How much do I have to do, and how hard do I have to do it? The answer, of course, depends on your individual fitness level and what your goals are; however, I think that there are some basic rules that all of you, no matter where you are or where you're going, should be aware of. So let me address the question of duration and intensity as well as what's the best type of aerobic exercise. This will also give me a chance to clear up some perpetual misconceptions about aerobic workouts.

- *How often do I need to do aerobic exercise?* That's a simple enough question—so why have there been so many different answers to it? Probably because this is one piece of the fitness puzzle that is inextricably tied to what your individual goals are. If your goal is to just be healthier, reduce your risk of disease, and keep your heart and lungs strong, you can get by with three days a week of aerobic exercise. But for the purposes of this program, where the goal is a total body makeover and an aggressive decrease in body fat, you need to engage in aerobic exercise six days a week. It doesn't always have to be the same workout—indeed, I hope you will vary your aerobic workouts, which will not only help you get better results but also help keep you safe from injury. And not all of you will be doing the same amount of minutes per session; that will depend on your fitness level. However, if you want to achieve a real transformation, you've got to get out there and do something aerobic almost every day.

- *How long do I need to exercise?* There has been a lot of talk about how fifteen minutes of aerobic exercise a session is all you really need. There's no doubt that fifteen minutes is better than nothing, but the truth is that if you want to accomplish more, you have to do more. If you're a beginner, I'm going to start you out slowly— and that may mean that you do only fifteen minutes per session (even less if that's all you're capable of). Everybody, from beginners to advanced, will tack 2 minutes on to their aerobic session each week. I'll also have you do one double-duration workout a week. This workout is meant to be done at a slightly slower pace, and its purpose is to build endurance. This slightly slower workout will help you burn some extra calories and give your muscles some time to recover from the faster-paced workouts so that you can come back stronger.

• *How hard do I have to exercise?* Intensity is an extremely important variable. With low-intensity exercise, you barely challenge your cardiovascular system or draw on your fuel reserves. Exercising at a moderately high intensity, however, does challenge your cardiovascular system, leading to significant physical changes, including an increase in your body's ability to perform aerobic work, a boost in metabolism both during and after exercise, and, most important, a reduction of body fat. If your goal is to make your body over as quickly as is reasonably possible, working out at a moderately high intensity is the way to go.

Let's talk about fat burning for a minute. For several years now, there has been widespread misunderstanding about the benefits of low- versus moderate- or high-intensity workouts. You may have heard that in order to burn fat, you need to exercise longer at a lower intensity. Technically, there's some truth to that. When you exercise at an easier pace (50 to 70 percent of your maximum ability), your body relies for its fuel on a higher percentage of stored fat calories than stored carbohydrate calories. Since fat is what you want to get rid of, it would seem that exercising at a lower intensity (between 50 and 70 percent of your maximum ability) is desirable. But the truth is that it doesn't matter whether you're burning fat or carbohydrate during your aerobic workout. What *does* matter is that you challenge your aerobic ability, which will cause the changes in your body necessary to increase your metabolism. This is what leads to dramatic body fat loss. **In order to increase your metabolic rate substantially, you need to work out vigorously.**

What's "vigorously"? Exercising in what's called "the zone." There are two ways to determine if you're in the zone. One requires measuring your heart rate; the other requires measuring how you feel. Here are the particulars of both methods, along with the pros and cons of each:

Your Target Heart Rate Range

Using some calculations involving your age and a formula developed by fitness experts, it's possible to figure out the number of beats per minute your heart will produce when you're exercising at your maximum ability. If, for instance, you're 40 years old, 100 percent of your maximum beats per minute (bpm) will be estimated at 180. No one, even elite athletes, exercises at the maximum for an extended period of time. Instead, for the best training effect, what you want to do is work out at a pace that's between 70 and 80 percent of your maximum ability. That target heart rate range is what's known as the zone. Here's how you figure it out:

220 – Your age x .70 = The lower limit of your target heart rate range
220 – Your age x .80 = The upper limit of your target heart rate range

Thus, for a 40-year-old, the range would be 126 bpm (220 – 40 x .70) to 144 bpm (220 – 40 x .80).

Once you know these numbers, you can take your pulse during your workout (wait until you're at least five minutes into it) and gauge whether or not you're in the zone. Keeping track of your heart rate range will ensure that you're exercising hard enough to make a difference. It's also provides a very tangible way to monitor your improvement. As you get fitter, you'll see that it takes a lot more effort to get your heart rate numbers up—a sign that your body is adapting to the exercise and you're getting into better shape. For instance, at the start of this program a 40-year-old beginner might reach 126 bpm just by walking at 3.5 mph on the treadmill. A month or two later, she might have to speed it up to 4.5 mph to be able to hit 126. But no matter what level you are, after 12 weeks on this program, your numbers are likely to clue you into how much you've improved.

While I'm not against using this method of determining whether you're exercising in the zone, there is a downside: it's not always easy to take your pulse during exercise. The ideal way to use this method is to get a heart rate monitor. The best of these monitors use a strap worn around your chest, which transmits your heart rate to a watchlike device. They're fairly easy to use and are reasonably accurate.

But even with the heart rate monitor, this method can still be an imperfect gauge of intensity. Heart rate doesn't always directly reflect how hard you're working or how much oxygen you're consuming. A number of other factors—your emotional state, medications you're taking, the temperature and altitude where you are, your caffeine consumption, to name a few—can alter your heart rate beyond the effects of exercise, throwing the whole equation off. Moreover, the formula itself is imperfect. Some estimate that it's accurate for only about one third of the population.

Personally, I think that the second method of determining if you're in the zone, perceived exertion, is preferable for most people. Try both, and see which one works best for you.

Perceived Exertion

How hard do you *think* you're working? That's the basic idea behind this method of monitoring intensity. To answer the question, you mainly take note of your breathing, your degree of muscle fatigue, and your general feeling of discomfort, then rate your overall state on a scale of 0 to 10. Zero is how it feels to be at rest; 10 is an exertion level so difficult that you could probably maintain it for only a few seconds (think back on when you had to do the fifty-yard dash in school—that gasping breathing, pitter-pattering heart, and burning muscles indicate a ten). The zone, according to this scale, is 7 or 8. At level 7, you feel as though your body is working fairly hard but also feel that you can maintain the pace for the rest of your workout. Your breathing is deep, but you can still carry on a conversation. Level 8 is slightly more vigorous. You might not be 100 percent sure that you'll be able to keep up the pace for the entire workout, and while you can still carry on a conversation, you probably wouldn't want to. Your optimum level is anywhere between 7 and 8, though most of you will probably start out at a 7 and work your way up to an 8.

If you're a beginner, it may take you a while to maintain level 7 consistently, but don't be discouraged. If you can't exercise at that pace for your whole workout, start at a lower level of exertion, then increase to 7 for 1 or 2 minutes at a time. Probably within a week or two you'll be able to exercise at level 7 for at least 10 to 15 minutes. Remember that highly aerobic exercise isn't supposed to be completely comfortable. You need to challenge yourself if you want to see some results.

Read the specifics of each level to get a sense of what's too much, too little, and just right.

PERCEIVED EXERTION
What You Should Be Feeling at Each Level

0: This is the feeling you would experience at rest. There is no feeling of fatigue. Your breathing is not at all elevated. You will not experience this level during exercise.

1: This is the feeling you would experience while working at your desk or reading. There is no feeling of fatigue. Your breathing is not elevated.

2: This is the feeling you would experience while getting dressed. There is little or no feeling of fatigue. Your breathing is not elevated. You will rarely experience this low level during exercise.

3: This is the feeling you would experience while slowly walking across the room to turn on the television. There is little feeling of fatigue. You may be slightly aware of your breathing, but it is slow and natural. You may experience this right at the beginning of an exercise session.

4: This is the feeling you would experience while slowly walking outside. There is a very slight feeling of fatigue. Your breathing is slightly elevated but comfortable. You should experience this level during the initial stages of your warmup.

5: This is the feeling you would experience while walking to the store. There is a slight feeling of fatigue. You are aware of your breathing, which is deeper than that of level 4. You should experience this level at the end of your warmup.

6: This is the feeling you would experience when you are walking to an appointment and are very late. There is a general feeling of fatigue, but you know that you can maintain this level of exertion. Your breathing is deep, and you are aware of it. You should experience this level in the transition from your warmup to your exercise session and during the initial phase of learning how to work at level 7 or 8.

7: This is the feeling you would experience while exercising vigorously. There is a definite feeling of fatigue, but you are quite sure you can maintain this level for the rest of your exercise session. Your breathing is deep, and you are definitely aware of it. You could carry on a conversation, but you would probably choose not to do so. This is the baseline level of exercise that you should maintain in your workout sessions.

8: This is the feeling you would experience when you are exercising *very* vigorously. There is a definite feeling of fatigue, and if you asked yourself if you could continue for the remainder of your exercise session, your answer would be that you think you could but you're not 100 percent sure. Your breathing is very deep. You could still carry on a conversation, but you wouldn't feel like it. This is the feeling you should experience only after you are comfortable reaching level 7 and are ready for a more intense workout. This is the level that produces rapid results for many people.

9: This is the feeling you would experience if you were exercising very, very vigorously. You would experience a definite feeling of fatigue, and if you asked yourself if you could continue the pace for the remainder of your exercise session, your answer would be that you probably could not. Your breathing is very labored. It would be very difficult to carry on a conversation. This is a feeling you may experience for short periods when trying to achieve a level 8. This is the level at which many athletes train, and it is difficult for them. You should not be experiencing level 9 on a routine basis and should slow up when you do.

10: You should not experience level 10. This is the feeling you would have with all-out exercise. This level cannot be maintained for very long, and there is no benefit in reaching it.

- **What kind of exercise?** Training the cardiovascular system requires aerobic (cardiovascular) exercise, the type of workout that causes your heart rate and breathing to accelerate. "Aerobic" simply means "with oxygen"; your muscles, when engaged in aerobic exercise, are primarily fueled by O_2. "Anaerobic" means "without oxygen" and is descriptive of another, oxygen-free metabolic process that the body uses to fuel the muscles during other types of exercise. Most workouts are not entirely aerobic or entirely anaerobic; however, exercise that you do at a pace you can sustain for a period of time—brisk walking, running, or cross-country skiing, for instance—are mostly aerobic. Workouts such as weight training and sprinting, which require quick, powerful efforts, are mostly anaerobic.
- **Choosing aerobic activities?** Just about anything that gets your heart rate up and allows you to sustain it for at least 20 minutes will help train your cardiovascular system to good effect. But if you hope to stick with your workout—remember how crucial consistency is— your chances will be better if you choose an activity that you like and

can readily do. Cycling, for instance, is great exercise, but not if you don't have any safe roads or paths you can ride on.

Even better, choose two or three activities. You could just let walking, for instance, be your only activity, but you will get into so much better shape if you expand your aerobic workout horizons. Mixing it up—called cross-training—will give you the best results for a couple of reasons. One is that it will reduce your risk of injury. If you do the same activity relentlessly day after day, you put a lot of stress on the same muscles and joints, increasing the chance that you may hurt yourself. Cross-training—particularly if you choose an activity that's considerably different than your primary one—gives your muscles a break and develops different areas of your body. Swimming, for instance, works your muscles differently from running and gives your joints some relief from the pounding. Running is a largely lower body activity; swimming relies more on the upper body. The more muscles you work, the fitter you're going to get. Cross-training also has another benefit: It will help keep you from getting burnt out. Doing the same thing day after day can get monotonous; I personally find that it's nice to have some variety.

All aerobic activities have value, but they're not all created equal. Activities that require you to support your own weight— such as walking and running—burn more calories than activities in which your weight is supported by, say, water or a bike. This isn't to say that supported activities such as cycling and swimming can't be done at a pace that makes them very high calorie burners. But most people don't swim laps or pedal a bike at that accelerated pace. (If you do, then by all means, let one of these workouts be your aerobic mainstay.)

I've developed a hierarchical chart of aerobic activities to guide you in making your workout choices. Again, all cardio workouts have value, but we're talking about a total body makeover in 12 weeks here. This is the time to take on something tough and work toward a big transformation.

SOME MEDICAL CAVEATS

It's absolutely imperative that you don't choose workouts that will compromise your health and safety. If you have high blood pressure, heart problems, or lung disease, are a smoker, or have any other serious medical condition, check with your doctor first. You will probably need to stay away from the more vigorous activities. Likewise, consult your physician if you have any orthopedic problems. Certain activities, including those performed on exercise machines, can exacerbate muscle and joint aches and pains.

AEROBIC WORKOUTS

BEST	GOOD	OKAY
These workouts burn ample amounts of calories, are convenient, and aren't too easy or too hard.	These workouts can be equally as good as the "best" activities; however, they may not be as convenient or readily available.	These workouts are slightly less aerobic and sometimes problematic. Use them only as secondary activities.
Power walking: This is my number one choice because anyone can do it anywhere and the risk of injury is low. If you do it on a treadmill, you can even control the grade in order to make the workout more challenging.	Stair stepping: Here I'm referring to the stair-stepping machine. It provides a great workout as long as you maintain good posture (don't lean on the machine arms) and don't overdo it—too much stair stepping can be hard on the knees.	Jumping rope: If you're good at this and fit, it provides an excellent workout. However, it can get pretty tedious, and it can be tough on the body. For most beginners, jumping rope is simply too strenuous to maintain for a long time.

BEST	GOOD	OKAY
Running: This is perhaps the most perfect exercise in terms of challenging your cardiovascular system; however, its injury rate is much higher than that of walking and is not recommended if you have high blood pressure or heart problems. This may be a workout that you'll want to work up to as you get fitter.	Elliptical exercise: Elliptical machines can really get your heart rate up, and they do so with a minimum of impact. The best machines let you work both your arms and legs.	In-line skating: To make this an effective activity, you have to skate continuously, which can sometimes be hard to do if you don't have a good pathway to do it on. If you do choose this workout, be sure to wear protective gear.
Aerobic dance: These days "aerobics," as we once knew them, have all different kinds of names: cardio funk, hip hop, cardio salsa, African dance, kickboxing, the list goes on. As long as the class is dance- or marital arts–based, gets your heart rate up for an extended period of time, and is low-impact, go for it. (If, on the other hand, it's high-impact, pass unless you're already fit and not prone to injuries.) This is a really fun way to get in your aerobic minutes.	Spinning: This stationary cycling class can be very invigorating; the music is usually loud and the energy high, plus it's as easy as, well, riding a bike. You can also set your own pace (as opposed to an aerobic dance class, where you run the risk of someone crashing into you if you slow down).	Outdoor rowing: If you have the equipment, rowing can be ideal. It works both the upper and lower body without a lot of stress, and gliding on water is a wonderful feeling. I'm putting it in the "Okay" column only because most people can't do it on a regular basis.
Stair climbing: Walking briskly or jogging up and down stairs can be strenuous, and you have to have the knees for it (anyone with orthopedic or heart problems should probably skip	Stationary cycling; You'll probably work harder in a spinning class than you will on a stationary bike by yourself. However, this can be a very convenient and effective way to get	

BEST

it), but it's also a convenient efficient workout. You may have to build up to where you can go continuously for 10 minutes before you can adopt it as your main or secondary activity.

GOOD

your cardiovascular workout in. Just be sure you maintain the proper intensity with this exercise.

OKAY

"Half" workouts: Because their contribution to weight loss is minimal, you get credit for only half the time spent participating in the following activities.

Indoor rowing: This activity is one of the few that works both your arms and legs. Plus you're not likely to injure yourself—it's virtually nonimpact. As with stationary cycling, though, it's easy to slack off, so make sure you get into the zone as you row.

Recumbent cycling: If you have a back problem, this supported style of stationary cycling can be a good choice. But it can also be performed with little effort, which is why I don't recommend it for weight loss.

Indoor cross-country skiing: Like rowing, it trains your arms and legs. This machine seems to have lost a little ground in gyms, but if you can find it, it's a worthwhile apparatus.

Swimming: The fact that swimming is nonimpact is in its favor: the problem with swimming is that unless you do it really vigorously, it doesn't allow your body to heat up the way other types of aerobic exercise do. When you heat up, you usually experience a decrease in appetite; swimming can actually increase your appetite. Plus if you're carrying a lot of body fat, you'll be fairly buoyant so your body won't have to work so hard to move through the water, thus decreasing your calorie-burning potential.

BEST	GOOD	OKAY
	Outdoor cycling: This can be a great option if you live close to safe, open roads or bike paths—and if you work hard and not just pedal along dreamily. I'd skip it, though, if you don't have a good place to ride.	Recreational sports: Tennis, basketball, volleyball, softball . . . I encourage you to participate in these and other fun sports. I want you not to just work out but to have an active life, and these can contribute to that. But remember, the time spent playing a sport counts for only half.

Strength Training

Considering what we now know about the value of strength training, it's hard to believe that it was once almost exclusively practiced by body builders and gym rats. Today we know that it's important for everyone, men and women alike, to strength train, and for a number of reasons. Even if you are already lifting weights and know something about how strength training changes the body, don't skip this section before you go on to the exercises.

Usually, when we think about our muscles, we think about strength—or the lack thereof. How strong you are defines your ability to "move resistance." In other words, how well can you push something away from you, pull something toward you, or lift something up? But strength isn't all that matters when it comes to muscles. To be able to accomplish what you need them to, your muscles also need power and endurance. "Power" refers to your muscles' ability to move resistance quickly, "endurance" refers to their ability to perform the work for extended periods of time. The weight-training exercises you'll be doing throughout the Total Body Makeover program address all three qualities: strength, power, and endurance.

Many people, as they age, seem to lose all facets of muscle potency. What they're *really* losing is muscle tissue, and mostly because they haven't challenged their muscles in any significant way. This is really a case of "use it or lose it": if you don't use it, you'll lose not only strength, power, and endurance but some of your calorie-burning potential as well. Muscle is the most calorie-hungry tissue in the body; maintaining it uses about four times the amount of calories that maintaining fat does. Strength training can do wonders to reverse muscle loss, even if you have never touched a weight or have not picked one up in years. In fact, some research suggests that you can reverse two decades of muscle loss in just eight weeks if you strength train conscientiously. Not incidentally, strength training with weights also helps build bone, lowering your risk of osteoporosis, and increases the body's ability to use insulin to clear sugar from the blood, reducing the risk of diabetes.

Weight training, of course, is also going to make a difference in the way you look. Over time, it will reduce the amount of body fat you're carrying and, as a result, reduce your overall size. Strengthening exercises also give the muscles definition, so that your body looks fitter and trimmer. It does not, in most cases, make women develop a bulky, masculine build. Unless you are a body builder who has an extreme training program and follows a muscle-building diet, you're not going to bulk up very much.

When you strength train, the exertion creates microtears in the muscle tissue. Think of it as "creative destruction": the tears stimulate the body to repair itself, and the repairs create larger, denser, and stronger muscles. This tear-and-repair scenario also helps activate nerves within the muscles that allow them to respond to challenges better. In addition, the process increases certain enzymes in the muscles, improving the way the body uses oxygen and fuel.

There's a fairly obvious way to determine if your muscles are adequately responding to strength training: muscle soreness—you should feel it. The discomfort shouldn't be so great that you find it hard to walk or open a door, but some soreness the next day lets you know your workouts are working. Often people—and certainly you intermediate and advanced exercisers are candidates—feel more discomfort 48 hours after a very hard workout, so if you feel sorest two days postlifting, don't be alarmed. It's a sign that you're working hard and improving.

Strength training and cardiovascular exercise are completely different activities. Many people consider them to be interchangeable, but that's a mistake. While there may be some benefit overlap, in the big picture they accomplish very different goals. You cannot build your cardiovascular system sufficiently with strength training alone. Likewise, you cannot build your muscles sufficiently with cardiovascular workouts alone—ask any professional athlete, most of whom combine the two types of exercise for optimal performance.

It's also important to remember that if you hope to see the toned, shapely muscles developed by strength training, you will have to burn the fat that lies on top of them. Strength training will improve your calorie burning throughout the day, but it's the extended cardiovascular workout, along with eating in moderation, that's really going to help you burn a sizable number of calories and shed excess pounds. So while it's fine to perform both strength training and a cardio workout in one session, it's not okay to substitute one for the other.

Like the effects of cardiovascular exercise, the effects of strength training depend on a few different variables. Here is what you need to know about each of them.

- **How many repetitions should you do?** Each time you raise and lower (or push against and retreat from) a resistance, or each time you curl up and down when doing an abdominal exercise, you've performed a repetition. What many people haven't figured out yet about repetitions is how many they should do. I'm often asked, "Isn't it best to do as many repetitions as possible?" The answer is yes—and no.

    First, the number of repetitions you'll be able to do will depend on the amount of resistance—i.e., how heavy the weight—you're working with. A lower level of resistance will allow you to do a higher number of repetitions, and a higher number of repetitions, in general, builds muscular endurance more than muscular strength. If, on the other hand, you use a heavier weight and do a lower number of repetitions, you will build some endurance but will largely be rewarded with more muscular strength. Because I think it's best to develop a combination of both endurance and strength, the ideal strength-training plan for a body makeover falls in the middle of high and low repetitions: 8 to 10 per set. I also like these numbers because they work well as a compliment to aerobic exercise. When you're engaged in a cardio workout, you're already building some muscular endurance by, say, swinging your arms when you walk or repeatedly moving your quads and hamstrings on the elliptical trainer. For core exercises, such as abdominals, I recommend a higher number of repetitions: 15 per set, with advanced exercisers even working up to as many as 40 or even 50 repetitions for some specialty exercises. Since you use your core muscles to stabilize your body all day long, endurance is a critical factor in determining their fitness. This is the perfect case when a higher number of repetitions makes sense.

- **How many sets should you do?** By organizing your repetitions (or reps, as they're usually called) into sets, you'll be able to do more of them and ultimately enhance the degree of fatigue in your muscles. That fatigue, in turn, will enhance the training effect. If you're a beginner, start with only 1 or 2 sets per exercise, then build up to 3 sets when you feel you can. When you start adding sets, you may not be able to do as many repetitions as you did in the previous set. Say, for instance, you do one set of 10 but find, in the second set, that you can reach only seven reps before you can go no further. That's perfectly fine; in fact, it's evidence that your muscles are becoming fatigued enough to get stronger. It's when everything comes too easily that you'll want to make adjustments, which I'll tell you more about when I talk about progressing.

- **How heavy should your weights be?** I wish I had simple numbers I could give you to help you choose the appropriate weights. But it's different for everybody, different for different exercises, and, as you become fitter, will even differ from the weights you used a few weeks before. However, I have a method for choosing weights that

I think works pretty well. Start with very light resistance, then go up to the next size weight, and, through trial and error, find the weights that make your muscles feel fatigued after lifting them 8 to 10 times. And by fatigued I mean that you can barely accomplish the last repetition. You don't want weights that are too heavy, but neither do you want ones that are too light. Another way you can tell if you're using the right amount of weight is if you feel slightly sore a day or two after training. You shouldn't feel so sore and uncomfortable that you want to skip your workouts. If that's the case, lighten the weights you're using.

- **How long should you rest between sets?** Rest in between sets is important; it allows you ultimately to do more repetitions than if you just kept on going without a break. However, I often see people taking too long between sets, and that can really impact the effectiveness of your training. Extended rest makes strength training easier, but it also lessens the strength-building fatigue effect, so don't take more than 15 to 30 seconds of rest between sets. As a general guideline, beginners can rest 30 seconds; intermediate exercisers, 20 to 25 seconds; and advanced exercisers, 15 seconds. Take even a shorter break between sets—about 5 seconds, the time it takes to take a deep breath—when doing abdominal exercises. Also, if you're doing an exercise that requires lifting first on one side, then on the other, do *all* the sets on one side before moving on to the second side. Don't alternate between sides, because, again, you don't want the muscles you're working to get too much rest.

  At first you may find that resuming an exercise quickly will make it impossible for you to do as many repetitions as you did the first set. That's okay; it's proof that your workout is producing the desired effect.

- **Should you use free weights or weight machines?** Both. I really like dumbbells, especially for beginners, and most of the exercises in the program are done with dumbbells. You don't have to commit to a gym; you can just go to the store, pick up a few sets of weights, and you're off and running. But a few of the intermediate and advanced exercises require the use of weight machines. None of the exercises calls for very exotic machines; you should be able to find them at even the most basic gym. You can, in fact, do most of the exercises on weight machines if you prefer. Since machines vary from place to place, I suggest that you get one of the trainers or managers at your gym to give you a lesson on how to use the machines properly. Most gyms offer this service for no extra charge.

- **How often should you exercise?** If you're aiming for optimal results, strength train three times a week; better-seasoned exercisers should do so every other day. Research has shown that you can strength train as infrequently as once a week and still maintain your current level of muscular strength and endurance. Twice a week will give you slight improvements. But I say go for three. It gives you the best results. Strength training really doesn't take much time (especially if you watch those between-set breaks!), so why not do the best you can?

The Exercises

Equipment needs: Dumbbells of various weights, a barbell (optional), a bench, and access to weight machines (for intermediate and advanced exercisers). Exercises designed especially for weight machines are indicated by an asterisk.

Beginner—Advanced: The Basic Eight

1. Squats

Target area: Upper legs (quadriceps, hamstrings)

The setup: Stand with your feet slightly wider than shoulder width apart, your back straight, your head up, and your toes and knees pointed slightly out. There should be a slight bend in your knees. Hold a dumbbell in each hand, your arms at your sides and your palms facing inward.

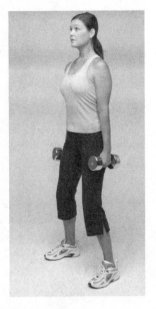

Starting position

The move: Contract your abdominal muscles, bend your knees, and gradually lower your body until your thighs are almost parallel with the floor. Never let them go past parallel with the floor. Control your movement through the entire exercise, inhaling on the way down and exhaling on the way up. Pause for a second, then push up from your heels and gradually return to the starting position. Continue until the entire set of 8 to 10 repetitions is complete. If you are performing multiple sets of this exercise, take a deep breath, wait 15 to 30 seconds, and begin your next set.

Tip: Be sure your torso is leaning forward only slightly throughout the exercise.

Weight machine alternative: Leg press machine

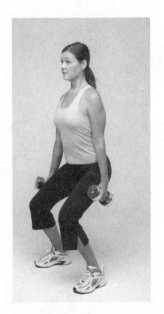

Active phase

2. Lunges

Target area: Legs (quadriceps, hamstrings, calves)

The setup: Stand with your feet shoulder width apart, your back straight, your head up, and your knees slightly bent. Hold a dumbbell in each hand, your arms at your sides and your palms facing inward.

The move: Contract your abdominal muscles. Step forward with your right foot and bend both knees so that your front thigh becomes parallel to the floor. Your front knee should be directly above your ankle—never beyond it. Pause for a second, then return to the starting position by pushing off from your front foot. Control your movement throughout the exercise, inhaling as you step forward and exhaling on the return. Continue until the entire set of 8 to 10 repetitions is complete. Switch sides. If you are performing multiple sets of this exercise, take a deep breath, wait 15 to 30 seconds, and begin your next set.

Tip: Keep your torso erect throughout the entire exercise.

No weight machine alternative

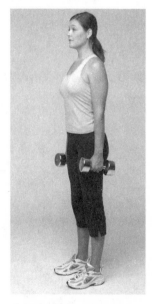

Starting position

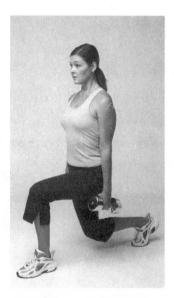

Active phase

3. Chest Press

Target area: Chest and back of upper arms (pectoralis major, pectoralis minor, triceps)

The setup: Lie on your back on a bench with your knees bent, feet flat on the floor. Keep your back flat against the bench with little or no arch. Hold a dumbbell in each hand slightly above chest level, palms facing forward.

The move: Contract your abdominal muscles. Gradually raise both dumbbells up until your arms are fully extended above your chest. Do not hyperextend your elbows. Pause for a second, then gradually return the dumbbells back to the starting position. Control your movements throughout the exercise, exhaling while raising the dumbbells and inhaling on the return. Continue until the entire set of 8 to 10 repetitions is complete. If you are performing multiple sets of this exercise, take a deep breath, wait 15 to 30 seconds, and begin your next set.

Tips: Keep your head and back firmly against the bench throughout the entire exercise. If lying on the bench with your feet on the floor is hard on your back, you can bend your knees and place your feet on the bench.

Weight machine alternative: Chest press machine

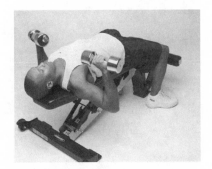

Active phase

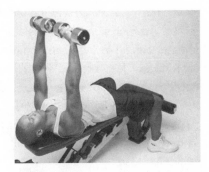

Starting position

4. Shoulder Press

Target area: Shoulders

The setup: Sit upright on a chair (or slightly slanted if you're using an incline bench) with your back supported and your feet flat on the floor. Keep your back flat against the back of the chair with little or no arch. Hold a dumbbell in each hand, slightly above shoulder level and with your palms facing forward, elbows out to the side.

The move: Contract your abdominals. Keeping your palms facing forward, raise the dumbbells up and inward until the inside ends of the dumbbells are nearly touching each other and are directly overhead. Do not hyperextend your elbows. Pause for a second, then gradually lower the dumbbells to the starting position. Control your movements throughout the exercise, exhaling while raising the dumbbells and inhaling on the return. Continue until the entire set of 8 to 10 repetitions is complete. If you are performing multiple sets of this exercise, take a deep breath, wait 15 to 30 seconds, and begin your next set.

Tip: Keep your back firmly against the chair or incline bench throughout the entire exercise.

Weight machine alternative: Shoulder press machine

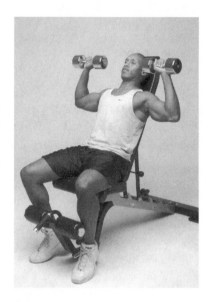

Starting position

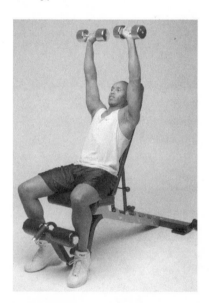

Active phase

5. Butterfly

Target area: Upper back (trapezius, latissimus dorsi)

The setup: Sit upright on a chair with your back supported and your feet flat on the floor. Keep your back flat against the back of the chair with little or no arch. Hold a dumbbell in each hand, slightly above shoulder level and with your palms facing forward, forearms parallel to each other in front of your chest. Keep your forearms about 4 or 5 inches apart and your elbows pressed against the front of your body.

The move: Contract your abdominals. Contract the muscles of your upper back while you rotate your shoulders back in a semicircle, bringing your elbows out to the side. Keep both dumbbells above shoulder height throughout the exercise. Pause for a second, then gradually return to the starting position. Control your movements throughout the exercise, exhaling while rotating the dumbbells and inhaling on the return. Continue until the entire set of 8 to 10 repetitions is complete. If you are performing multiple sets of this exercise, take a deep breath, wait 15 to 30 seconds, and begin your next set.

Tips: Keep your head straight up while looking forward and your back straight throughout the entire exercise. To do the rotation correctly, it's helpful to visualize squeezing something like a piece of paper between your shoulder blades and holding it for a split second.

Weight machine alternative: Upright rowing machine

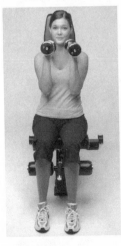 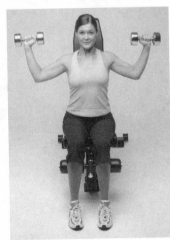

Starting position   *Active phase*

6. Dumbbell Fly

Target area: Chest (pectoralis major, pectoralis minor)

The setup: Lie on your back on a bench with your knees bent, feet flat on the floor. Keep your back flat against the bench with little or no arch. With your arms fully extended (but not hyperextended) above your chest, hold a dumbbell in each hand, palms facing inward.

The move: Contract your abdominal muscles. Gradually lower the dumbbells out to the side, keeping your elbows slightly bent throughout the entire exercise. Continue until your upper arms are parallel with the floor. Pause for a second, then gradually return to the starting position. Control your movements throughout the entire exercise, exhaling while lowering the dumbbells and inhaling on the return. Continue until the entire set of 8 to 10 repetitions is complete. If you are performing multiple sets of this exercise, take a deep breath, wait 15 to 30 seconds, and begin your next set.

Tips: Keep your head and back firmly against the bench throughout the entire exercise. If lying on the bench with your feet on the floor is hard on your back, you can bend your knees and place your feet on the bench.

Weight machine alternative: Fly machine

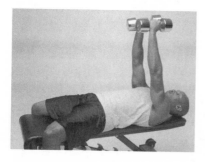

Starting position

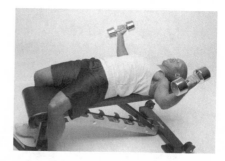

Active phase

7. Biceps Curl

Target area: Upper arms (biceps)

The setup: Stand with your feet slightly apart and your knees slightly bent. Hold a dumbbell in each hand using an underhand grip, your arms at your sides, palms facing inward.

The move: Contract your abdominals. Curl the dumbbells up to your shoulder while twisting your palms so that they are facing you at the top of the move. Pause for a second, then gradually lower the dumbbells to the starting position. Control your movements throughout the entire exercise, exhaling while lifting the dumbbells up and inhaling on the return. Continue until the entire set of 8 to 10 repetitions is complete. If you are performing multiple sets of this exercise, take a deep breath, wait 15 to 30 seconds, and begin your next set.

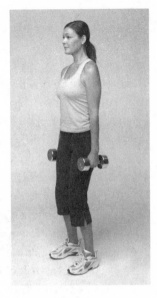

Starting position

Tip: Maintain your posture throughout the entire exercise and do not allow the dumbbells to "fall" back down.

Weight machine alternative: Curl machine

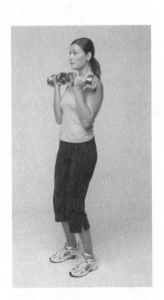

Active phase

8. Triceps Extension

Target area: Back of upper arms (triceps)

The setup: Stand with your feet slightly apart and your knees slightly bent. With your arms fully extended (but not hyperextended) above your head, hold one dumbbell, using an interlocking grip.

The move: Contract your abdominal muscles. Gradually lower the dumbbell back behind your head and neck while keeping your elbows in place above your head. Continue until your forearms are parallel to the floor. Pause for a second, then gradually raise the dumbbell to the starting position. Control your movements throughout the entire exercise, inhaling while lowering the dumbbell and exhaling while raising it back up. Continue until the entire set of 8 to 10 repetitions is complete. If you are performing multiple sets of this exercise, take a deep breath, wait 15 to 30 seconds, and begin your next set.

Tip: Maintain your posture throughout the entire exercise; avoid arching your back.

Weight machine alternative: Triceps extension machine or cable pull

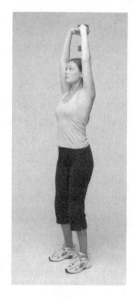

Starting position

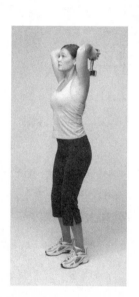

Active phase

Intermediate–Advanced

9. One-Arm Row

Target area: Back and shoulders

The setup: Kneel on a bench with your right arm supporting your weight. Hold a dumbbell in your left hand with your arm hanging down naturally, palm facing inward.

The move: Contract your abdominal muscles. Bend your left elbow and gradually raise the dumbbell to about chest height. Your elbow should be kept high and finish above your shoulder. Pause for a second, then return to the starting position. Control your movements throughout the entire exercise, exhaling as you raise the dumbbell and inhaling as you return to the starting position. Continue until the entire set of 8 to 10 repetitions is complete. Switch sides. If you are performing multiple sets of this exercise, take a deep breath, wait 15 to 30 seconds, and begin your next set.

Tip: Keep your back straight throughout the exercise.

Weight machine alternative: Upright Rowing Machine

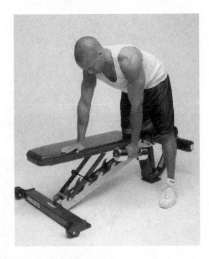
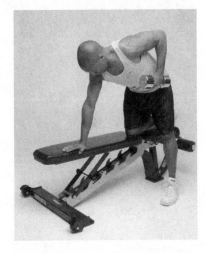

Starting position   *Active phase*

10. Lateral Raise

Target area: Shoulder/rotator cuff

The setup: Stand erect with your feet shoulder width apart, your arms down, and a slight bend in your elbows. Hold a dumbbell in each hand, one in front of each thigh, with your palms facing inward toward each other. Keep your knees slightly bent.

The move: Contract your abdominal muscles. Raise both dumbbells out to the sides in a semicircular motion. Pause for a second before gradually lowering the dumbbells to the starting position. Control your movements throughout the entire exercise, exhaling as you raise the dumbbells and inhaling as you return to the starting position. Continue until the entire set of 8 to 10 repetitions is complete. If you are performing multiple sets of this exercise, take a deep breath, wait 15 to 30 seconds, and begin your next set.

Tip: Keep your back straight and your head up as you go through the move.

Weight machine alternative: Lateral raise machine

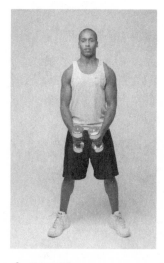

Starting position

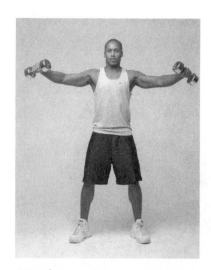

Active phase

11. Leg Press*

Target area: Quadriceps

The setup: On the leg press machine, select a seat setting that allows you to extend your legs fully. Your body should be erect, with your back firmly against the seat, and your feet should be squared or turned slightly outward, with the weight on the balls of your feet. Flex your knees at 90 degrees or less.

The move: Contract your abdominal muscles. Extend your legs completely, without locking your knees. Pause for a second, then return to the starting position. Pause for a second before starting the next repetition. Control your movements throughout the entire exercise, exhaling as you extend your legs and inhaling as you return to the starting position. Continue until the entire set of 8 to 10 repetitions is complete. If you are performing multiple sets of this exercise, take a deep breath, wait 15 to 30 seconds, and begin your next set.

Tip: The extension should take 2 to 3 seconds, as should the return to the starting position.

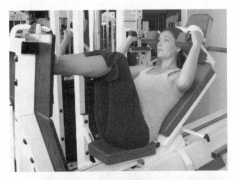

Starting position

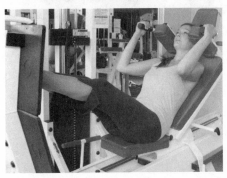

Active phase

12. Leg Extension*

Target area: Quadriceps

The setup: Adjust the leg arm of the leg extension machine so that your knees are centered with the pivot point. The leg pad should be adjusted so that it rests comfortably above the feet. Your body should be erect, with your back firmly against the seat. With your thighs parallel to each other and 4 to 5 inches of space between your knees, your legs straight but not locked, point your toes straight up or with a slight pitch forward. Grasp the handholds firmly and look straight ahead.

The move: Contract your abdominal muscles. Extend your legs completely without locking your knees. Pause for a second before returning the weight to the starting position. Pause for a second before starting the next repetition. Control your movements throughout the entire exercise, exhaling as you extend your legs and inhaling as you return to the starting position. Continue until the entire set of 8 to 10 repetitions is complete. If you are performing multiple sets of this exercise, take a deep breath, wait 15 to 30 seconds, and begin your next set.

Tip: The extension should take 2 to 3 seconds, as should the return to starting position.

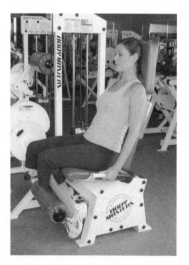

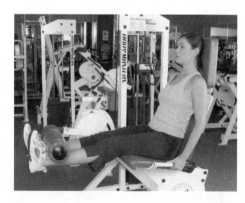

Active phase

Starting position

13. Leg Curl*

Target area: Hamstrings

The setup: Adjust the leg arm of the leg curl machine so that your knees are centered at the pivot point. The leg pad should be adjusted so that it rests comfortably on the back of the leg, just above the Achilles tendon. With your thighs parallel to each other and 4 to 5 inches of space between your knees, legs straight but not locked, point your toes up or with a slight pitch forward. Grasp the handholds firmly and look straight ahead.

The move: Contract your abdominal muscles. Bend your knees up to a 90-degree angle. Pause for a second, then allow your legs to come slowly back to the starting position. Pause for a second before starting the next repetition. Control your movements throughout the entire exercise, exhaling as you bend your legs and inhaling as you return to the starting position. Continue until the entire set of 8 to 10 repetitions is complete. If you are performing multiple sets of this exercise, take a deep breath, wait 15 to 30 seconds, and begin your next set.

Tip: The downward phase should take 2 to 3 seconds, as should the return to the starting position.

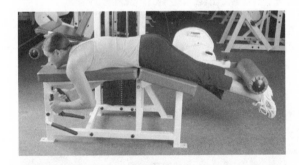

Starting position

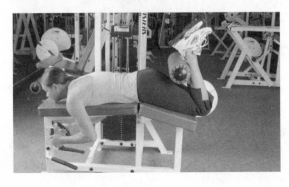

Active phase

14. Incline Press

Target area: Upper chest, back of upper arms

The setup: Lie with your back flat against an incline bench with little or no arch in your back. Keep your knees bent and your feet flat on the floor. Bend your elbows and hold a dumbbell in each hand slightly above chest level, palms facing forward.

The move: Contract your abdominal muscles. Gradually raise both dumbbells up until your arms are fully extended above your chest. Do not hyperextend your elbows. Pause for a second, then gradually return the dumbbells to the starting position. Control your movements throughout the entire exercise, exhaling upon raising the dumbbells and inhaling on the return. Continue until the entire set of 8 to 10 repetitions is complete. If you are performing multiple sets of this exercise, take a deep breath, wait 15 to 30 seconds, and begin your next set.

Tip: Keep your head and back firmly against the bench throughout the entire exercise.

Weight machine alternative: Incline press machine

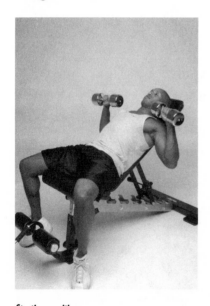 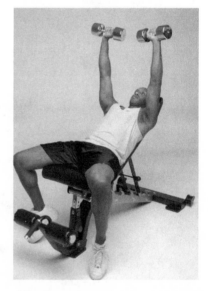

Starting position   *Active phase*

15. Upright Row

Target area: Shoulders (deltoids)

The setup: Stand with your feet shoulder width apart, your arms straight, and your torso erect. Using an overhand grip, hold a barbell or dumbbells in your hands, allowing them to rest lightly on your thighs (if using a barbell, grip the bar with your hands 2 to 4 inches apart).

The move: Contract your abdominal muscles. With your elbows pointed outward, gradually pull the weights upward along your abdomen and chest until your elbows reach shoulder height. Exhale as the weights reach your shoulders, pause for a second, and inhale as you gradually lower the weights to the starting position. Control your movements as you go. Continue until the entire set of 8 to 10 repetitions is complete. If you are performing multiple sets of this exercise, take a deep breath, wait 15 to 30 seconds, and begin your next set.

Tip: Keep your elbows higher than your wrists as you move the weights from the starting position to your shoulders.

Weight machine alternative: Upright rowing machine

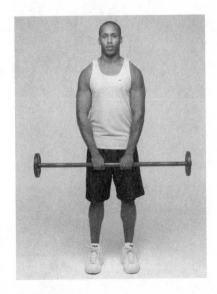

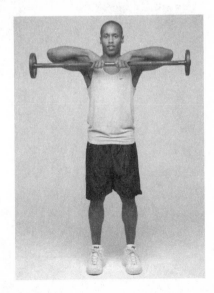

Starting position   *Active phase*

Advanced Only

16. Thumbs Down

Target area: Rotator cuff of the shoulder

The setup: Stand erect with your feet shoulder width apart. Holding a dumbbell in each hand in front of your thighs, rotate your arms inward so that your thumbs face your thighs. Keep your knees slightly bent.

The move: Contract your abdominal muscles. With your arms straight (but not hyperextended), raise both dumbbells in front of you to shoulder height while keeping your thumbs down and your arms rotated inward. Pause for a second, then return to the starting position. Control your movements throughout the entire exercise, exhaling as you raise the dumbbells and inhaling on the way down. Continue until the entire set of 8 to 10 repetitions is complete. If you are performing multiple sets of this exercise, take a deep breath, wait 15 to 30 seconds, and begin your next set.

Tip: Keep your back straight and your head up as you go through the move.

No weight machine alternative

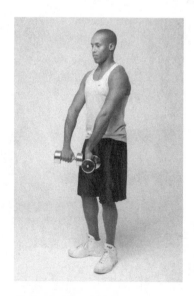

Starting position

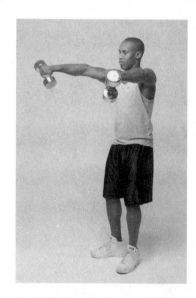

Active phase

17. Frontal Raise

Target area: Shoulders

The setup: Stand erect with your feet slightly apart. Hold a dumbbell in each hand with your arms down and your palms facing your thighs. Your closed fingers should be lightly touching your thighs. Keep your knees slightly bent.

The move: Contract your abdominal muscles. Raise both dumbbells in front of you to shoulder height. Pause for a second, then return to the starting position. Control your movements throughout the entire exercise, exhaling as you raise the dumbbells and inhaling on the way down. Continue until the entire set of 8 to 10 repetitions is complete. If you are performing multiple sets of this exercise, take a deep breath, wait 15 to 30 seconds, and begin your next set.

Tip: Keep your back straight and your head up as you go through the move.

No weight machine alternative

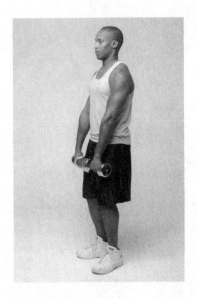
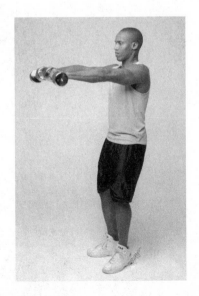

Starting position   *Active phase*

18. External Rotation

Target area: Shoulders/rotator cuff

The setup: Lie on a mat on your left side. Hold a dumbbell in your right hand, and bend your right arm at a 90-degree angle. Your elbow should rest against your side, slightly above your hip.

The move: Contract your abdominal muscles. Slowly raise the weight until it is pointed at the ceiling or as high as your range of motion allows. Pause for a second at the top before gradually lowering the dumbbell. Control your movements throughout the entire exercise, exhaling as you raise the dumbbell and inhaling on the way down. Continue until the entire set of 8 to 10 repetitions is complete. Switch sides. If you are performing multiple sets of this exercise, take a deep breath, wait 15 to 30 seconds, and begin your next set.

Tip: Keep your elbow close to your body as you lift and lower the weight.

No weight machine alternative

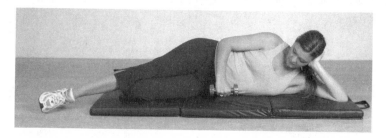

Starting position

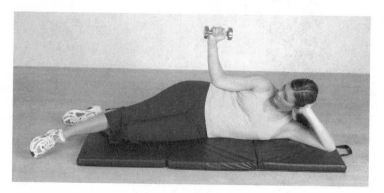

Active phase

19. Lat Pull-Down*

Target area: Upper back and chest muscles

The setup: While seated (or kneeling if the station has no seat) at a lat pull station, grip the bar using an overhand grip with your hands a few inches wider than shoulder width apart. Your torso should be slightly tilted backward and your arms extended.

The move: Contract your abdominal muscles. Pull the bar straight down in front of your face. Pull smoothly, keeping your elbows out and away from your body. Pull the bar past your chin until it lightly touches your upper chest. Pause for a second, then return to the starting position. Control your movements throughout the entire exercise, exhaling as the bar approaches your chest and inhaling as you release back to the starting position. Continue until the entire set of 8 to 10 repetitions is complete. If you are performing multiple sets of this exercise, take a deep breath, wait 15 to 30 seconds, and begin your next set.

Tip: Don't allow your back to arch as you pull down.

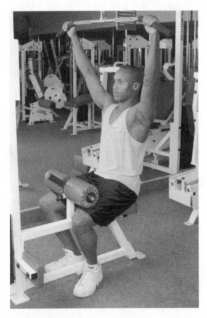
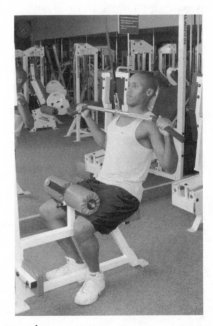

Starting position   *Active phase*

3

FIVE SIMPLE EATING RULES

THE EXERCISES YOU'LL BE doing during the next 12 weeks will help your body operate more efficiently and maximize the burning of calories. But there are also other things you can do to help ensure that optimal fat loss will occur. The five rules in this chapter sound simple—and they are—but that doesn't prevent them from having a big impact on many people's efforts to shape up. The level of impact, of course, will depend on what your eating habits are like now. If, for instance, you are a night eater (and I find that so many people are), the rule "Have an eating cutoff time" can cause big changes in your weight. Do you remember Shawn's story (page 35)? A chronic middle-of-the-night eater, she found that just following the cutoff rule was the first thing that really got some of the pounds to budge. Elizabeth (page 81) found that eliminating alcohol really helps her have more energy to exercise.

These rules are tested and true, and there's a good chance that they will be all you need, besides exercise, to transform yourself totally. In my experience working with clients, the vast majority of people who stick with them never need to go on a formal diet. The small percentage of those who don't respond completely can then opt to try a diet, which is an option for you as well at the end of the 12 weeks. If you're extremely impatient, you can even do so sooner, although I counsel patience—you may be surprised at how well you do with these five rules alone.

I should make it clear that despite the fact that I'm not asking you to follow a formal diet during this 12-week program, I do expect you to make an effort to choose healthful foods. The five rules I'm presenting here will help you do that, and so, indirectly, will the exercise program. Knowing that you have a demanding schedule ahead of you each day should give you the incentive to eat well. While overeating or bingeing on fatty, salty, and sugary foods will put a crimp in your ability to work out, consuming nutritious foods will give you the energy and nutrients you need to perform well. Avoid those foods, and you'll likely find yourself feeling sluggish and hard pressed to finish the activities you have committed yourself to. Exercise can make you feel great, but only if you support it with the proper fuel.

One of the most important rules is: Make eating a conscious act. What this mainly refers to is stopping emotional eating, a habit that undermines so many people's efforts to reshape their bodies. The definition of emotional eating is eating for emotional reasons and not due to true physical hunger. It may be a response to stress or boredom; to fill a void or soothe pain; to calm the mind or provide comfort in the face of fear, frustration, or regret. Emotional eating can even be eating to create a body that serves as a protective barrier, keeping others out both physically and emotionally.

If you are struggling with emotional eating, look at dealing with it as an opportunity for you to improve your life. Emotional eating is often not an eating *problem* as much as it is a *symptom* of other, larger problems. Look at the work you'll be doing to eliminate it as a blessing, because ultimately it's going to help you address the issues that are truly at the heart of your depression, anxiety, boredom, loneliness, or whatever it is that's making you turn to food for comfort.

Many people who eat for emotional reasons aren't even aware of it. But even if you do know what's driving you to consume food to mask your emotions, emotional eating is hard to shake. Food used this way is like a drug; it's addictive. And although there is no way you will ever alleviate your spiritual and emotional hunger by eating, giving up the habit can be a serious challenge.

Making a sincere attempt to do so now is important not only for your psychological well-being but because emotional eating can weaken your efforts to succeed in this 12-week program. Many times, when people who eat for emotional reasons succumb to a binge, they become so angry at themselves for indulging that they question why they're even trying to change their bodies. Unfairly, they take it as a confirmation that they don't deserve what it is they seek, and often they lose their resolve and end up quitting. Emotional eating can make you feel hopeless and incapable of doing the work necessary to create dramatic change. That's why it's so important to address emotional eating. The truth is, emotional eating isn't something that can typically be stopped overnight; you may, in fact, end up managing it more than vanquishing it completely.

The good news is that people do it. Successful people face up to the fact that they're eating for emotional reasons, and they make progress in limiting their emotional eating—and sometimes even eliminate it altogether. But perhaps most important, they identify what is making them turn to food, then call on their inner strength to alter the core aspect of their life that's driving the emotional eating. Even if they still find that they turn to food for comfort on occasion, they have gotten to the root of the problem, and that's what counts.

Eating consciously as well as following the other four simple eating rules may be just as critical to your success as every weight you lift and every minute you spend on your aerobic exercise. Put them onto your schedule as a reminder that you won't just be following an exercise prescription during the 12 weeks; you'll also be supporting your work-outs with healthy eating and drinking habits.

Breaking the Cycle of Emotional Eating
Dana's Story

When I was ten years old, my father died. Before that I was a tall, skinny kid. But after he died, people started offering me food as a kind of comfort, and eating soon became consolation. I yo-yoed up and down from a base of 160 to 165. At five feet, nine inches, I was a big girl but not obese. I went to college at 17 and gained not the "freshman ten," but the "freshman fifty."

I married Paul, my soul mate, when I was 24 and lost enough weight to wear a size 10—until I got pregnant a year later. I've never seen a pregnant woman so heavy. At Wal-Mart, people used to ask if I needed help getting back to my car!

I dropped down to 176 before getting pregnant with my second child and thought I looked good (now I cringe when I look at those photos!). But during that pregnancy I grew huge again, and I'm here to tell you that it's a myth that nursing takes the weight off.

In the autumn of 2001, I suffered back-to-back miscarriages. I was devastated. I'm a good mommy—that's what I do—and I'm proud of it. Losing those babies threw me for a loop. I started dealing with my dad's death again, and with that the emotional eating came back in full force. I ate chocolate all day long.

At the doctor's office in December 2002 I stepped on the scale and had a wake-up call. I weighed 248 pounds. I had degenerative discs that caused chronic back pain. I had TMJ, which caused headaches every single day. I was tired and sluggish all the time. And I was depressed.

I'm a Christian, and I thought, "This can't be the life I'm supposed to have." A few days later I was in Wal-Mart and I saw *O, The Oprah Magazine* with the blurb about Bob's book *The Get With the Program! Guide to Good Eating* and the challenge to lose weight and get healthy. I bought both. Even though I have two little girls and no time to read, I sat down and read the whole book, cover to cover, and decided to take up the challenge.

When I read Bob's words "Consider your health and well-being sacred. Don't let your obligations to others interfere with your obligations to yourself," it all clicked. Bob said of emotional eating, "You can break the cycle," I thought, "I can? But that's who I am, an emotional eater. That's what gets me through." Then I read, "If you're ready to change, you're ready to stop making excuses." At that moment, I said, "That's it! I'm done!" I turned around, faced everything, and I've never looked back.

I believed that if Jesus could save the world from sin, he could surely help me lose my rear end.

At 5 A.M. on the morning of January 2, 2003, while my family slept, I climbed onto my NordicTrack. At first I could only do fifteen minutes, I was so out of breath, but by the end of January I was going for an hour. Every day, no negotiations. I went to the grocery store with my list and with the book, recipes in hand. No more fat. No more sweets. And I drank all the water. Every day. I'd made up my mind, and I didn't want to do anything to sabotage my results.

Nobody said a word to me about my weight loss for the first two months, but I felt great—in fact, I felt better than I looked, and that was enough to keep me going. Eventually I added running, Rollerblading, and strength training to my workout. I get up early, I do it, and I feel bad if I don't. Not only do I eat a healthy diet, but so does my family, I'm teaching my daughters how to eat right so they don't have to struggle like I did.

My eyes now see the world differently. For the first time, I am comfortable with myself and my place in the world. I am healthier—no more back pain, no more headaches, no more sluggishness or depression. In fact, I am just giddy every morning when I wake up knowing I can work out, shower, and pull on a size 4 or 6 pair of jeans, (even shorts, for the first time ever). I have decided that the X on plus-size clothing stands for "expletive." I know I sure wanted to put one behind those numbers!

These days, I can wear a swimsuit without a cover-up—a bikini, in fact. I can see pride in my husband's and daughters' eyes as they introduce me. It's a wonderful feeling to be able to turn heads again, especially my husband's. My husband, who's known me since I was 18, looks at me differently now. One recent Sunday, when the girls were with their grandmother, he kept staring at me, and I asked, "What is it?" He actually had tears in his eyes when he said, "You look more beautiful than you ever have."

My little girls are proud of me, too, and it is an incredible feeling to know that I can be an example of health and fitness for their lives. One of the best moments of my life was when my oldest, Georgia Riley, who's 7 years old, put her arms around me with room to spare and said, "Look what I can do. This is my mom." I've changed not only my life, but my whole family's, too.

The Five Simple Eating Rules

1. Have an eating cutoff time.

Going to bed feeling a little hungry—a feeling of "Yeah, I could eat some-thing"—is a sign that your body is going to dip into its fat stores. All too often people give in to the urge to eat, and they miss this key opportunity to burn calories. The trick is just to get past that short period of discomfort.

Being able to go to bed with that tiny tug of hunger means that you're going to need to put some space between your final meal or snack and the time you head off to sleep. I don't mean that you should go to bed feeling really hungry or that everybody has to stop eating at 6 o'clock, a rule that is often imposed on dieters. But it does mean that you should stop eating at least two hours before bedtime. If you can hold out for three hours, even better. You can start with two hours and work your way up to two and a half, then three.

Although this rule is about *not eating,* it actually sets you up for a healthier pattern of eating. When you go to bed a little hungry, you'll also wake up hungry, and that means that you'll eat breakfast (see rule 2). That, in turn, will help maximize your calorie burning all day long. If, on the contrary, you eat right before you go to bed, hardly any of that food will be digested (digestion all but shuts down during sleep) and you won't want to eat for hours beyond the time you wake up.

There are other reasons why eating close to your shut-eye time can be disadvantageous. Although in general your metabolism speeds up every time you eat (the scientific name for it is the thermic effect), when you're close to going to sleep, your body is operating in slow gear—so slow that it might not even register the thermic effect. Plus, eating and then going to sleep gives you no time to work off the calories you've just taken in. As soon as you hit the pillow, you're going to burn only the bare minimum of calories you need to keep your basic body functions going. Had you con-sumed those same calories earlier, they probably would have increased your energy, causing you to move around more and thus burn more.

It's also not particularly healthy to go to sleep on a full stomach. As digestion shuts down during sleep, the food you've consumed has an extended contact time with your digestive tract. That increases your risk of various ailments and diseases, including certain cancers. Most people also feel pretty lousy when they go to bed soon after eating. Instead of feeling light and comfortable, they feel heavy and maybe even a little nauseous. In my mind, there's no contest. The former sounds a lot more appealing than the latter.

Most late-night eating is emotional eating, a salve at the end of the evening to cope with the dissatisfaction and disappointments of the day, or the dissatisfaction and disappointments of life in general. For that reason, having a cutoff time can be another tool in your arsenal to combat emotional eating. Another reason for night eating is mismanagement of your food intake during the day. If you didn't eat enough during the day, you're going to feel it at night. Don't skip meals (especially breakfast, which we'll get to next), and try to space out your meals and snacks so that you give your body what it needs throughout the day. Keep your meals moderate in size, neither overly large nor too skimpy. Treat your body right during the day, and you'll be far less likely to hit the fridge at night.

2. Eat a nourishing breakfast.

Many people simply aren't hungry in the morning, and, figuring that it gives them a painless way to eliminate calories, they see that as a sort of fortunate gift of nature. It would be if eating first thing in the morning didn't have such a positive effect on three factors that influence weight: your metabolism, your energy level, and how you eat during the rest of the day.

One thing we know about the metabolism is that it's at its lowest when you're asleep. You burn hardly any calories while you're snoozing. When you wake up in the morning, your metabolism begins to speed up, but slowly—unless you give it a boost. And that's what breakfast does.

Anytime you consume food, your body responds by raising the rate at which you burn calories (the thermic effect I mentioned before). That's useful no matter what time of day it is; however, in the morning the boost is particularly helpful because otherwise your body would still be operating in superlow gear. Essentially, what breakfast does is allow you to increase the number of hours your metabolism runs on high and, ultimately, the total amount of calories you burn in each 24-hour period. By the way, exercising in the morning also helps your body snap out of its postsleep, low-calorie-burning state. Exercise in the morning *and* eat breakfast, and you'll get a double whammy, increasing your metabolism even more—and more than if you did either one alone.

In most of the discussions about calorie burning and weight loss, the topic of how energetic a person feels hardly ever comes up, which I find surprising given that it's an important piece of the puzzle. If you feel energetic, you will move around more; the more you move around, the more calories you burn. I'm not talking about formal exercise per se, but rather all the little things you do during the day that contribute to your overall calorie burning. If you're feeling tired, will you take the stairs? Get up from your desk to talk to a colleague instead of just picking up the phone or e-mailing? Will you speed up to catch a bus or just resign yourself to waiting for the next one? Will you sit up attentively while talking to someone, instead of sinking lazily into the couch? My guess is no to all of the above.

Breakfast is your key to staying energized so that you *do* do all of those things. By elevating your blood sugar level, that morning meal will give you more get-up-and-go of both the physical and mental varieties. Think about all those studies that show that children do better in school when they eat breakfast than when they don't. The same is true for adults. Having a morning meal will improve your alertness and concentration. And it's so much easier to walk past the Danish-laden coffee cart when you're thinking straight and not weak and fatigued. Granted, if you've never been a breakfast eater, it can take some getting used to. It may take 5 to 6 weeks, but things will fall into place and you'll find that you actually wake up hungry in the morning.

Beyond that, eating breakfast can help you make better dietary decisions throughout the day. If you're a breakfast skipper, you're likely to be ravenous by the time lunch rolls around; that may cause you to overeat not only at lunch, but throughout the rest of the day. Research bears this out, showing that people who eat breakfast tend to consume fewer calories at lunch and dinner and snack less compulsively than people who don't take the time to eat in the morning. What's more, even though they consume fewer calories, breakfast eaters ultimately take in more vitamins and minerals than non–breakfast eaters.

Breakfast has so many benefits that it would be crazy not to take advantage of them. I hate to trot out an old cliché, but breakfast really is the most important meal of the day. So even if you have a lifelong habit of skipping the morning meal, now's the time to break it.

Faith, Friends, and Exercise Instead of Emotional Eating
Julie's Story

I have both college and graduate degrees, and I have had jobs that have given me a position of authority in the community. But my greatest accomplishment has been going from weighing 422 pounds, sitting on a couch in my southern hometown, to someone considerably lighter crossing the finish line of a half marathon in Anchorage, Alaska.

In high school I was voted Miss Personality by my schoolmates, though in reality I was crying the tears of a clown. I was already 250 pounds. By graduate school I hit 325 pounds and shortly thereafter was diagnosed with advanced melanoma. The doctors had to take out a portion of my calf and hip. I've been cancer-free now for 20 years.

After school I went to work as a magistrate, an initial appearance judge. People didn't take me seriously because of my weight. I had to do more to gain the same respect that was given to others who did less. From 1980 to 1990, I tried every form of weight loss gimmick and every diet known to man without permanent success. In 1991, I went to work in the DA's office. By this time I weighed in at 350 pounds, and I had a spiritual epiphany. I knew things needed to change. I knew deep down that I had never dealt with the old stuff in my life—specifically, the fact that I had been sexually abused by a neighbor as a child.

So I took some baby steps but I kept eating. I was feeding

my feelings, not feeling them. In 1996, I decided to seek the help of a therapist, but I couldn't face talking about the abuse. In the meantime, I had to have the top part of my spine rebuilt using my own hip bone and regenerated discs; then I had a pulmonary embolism that almost killed me. In 1997, I was diagnosed with lymphedema, a disease of the lymphatic system that causes severe fluid retention, and I had to spend a month in the hospital. This condition still causes my weight to fluctuate dramatically, but I have learned to cope with it.

Despite all this, my process of changing my life continued. I went back to therapy, and this time I knew there was no way around facing up to the problem. I cried a lot—I cried for a year!—about how much of my life I'd lost to being overweight. I called up my mother and said, 'Let's go to the YMCA and see if I can walk in the water.' I could, and I lost 40 pounds doing it. I still wasn't eating properly; I was on a lot of medications that made me nauseous, and I used that as an excuse to eat only ice cream and cheese and crackers. Though I cut back on the portion sizes, I didn't eat any healthier.

Finally, I went to Weight Watchers, where I learned how to eat healthfully. Now I was having a proper serving of cereal—¾ cup—not filling up the mixing bowl that I had been using before. The weight started moving off me rapidly, and at the same time I was gaining tools that I could use instead of food to meet my emotional needs: friends, exercise, and faith.

By now I'd lost 100 pounds, and when I decided I was ready to pump up the volume, a friend was kind enough to hire a personal trainer for me. And I'd thought therapy was torture! I showed up for the first workout wearing a flannel lumberjack shirt, spandex blue jeans, and hiking boots. The look on my trainer's face! I could see he was thinking, "Golly, I've got my work cut out for me." But both of us persevered. I learned to get on a treadmill and push through the discomfort. And I learned that the body can do a lot more than the mind says it can.

By this point I'd lost another 80 pounds. One day I saw a

brochure at the Y for a full and half marathon and thought, "Why not?" My sister encouraged me to go for it, and my best friend ran the race with me. I started training. I lost another 65 pounds, and I crossed the finish line. Not long before, I couldn't even walk far enough to get my mail. To me this just shows that there is hope, no matter what your challenges are.

My own experience led to me start a group program called HOPE—Helping Overweight People Embrace—which is now offered at many YMCAs. It deals with health and nutrition as well as the emotional issues behind being overweight. I know that I was eating to try to meet an emotional need that was never, ever going to be met by food. I now weigh about 175 pounds, though I still fluctuate, mostly due to the lymphedema. I'd like to get down to 140, but I also think, "Who cares? I used to weigh over 400 pounds!" My emotional issues have been resolved, I've found my wings, and I will continue to fly.

3. Drink a minimum of six 8-ounce glasses of water every day.

During the next 12 weeks, whether you're a beginner or an advanced-level exerciser, you're going to boost your activity level substantially, and that means you're going to need to drink a lot more water. You'll be losing water through perspiration at a time when it's critical for you to be adequately hydrated: your body can't cool itself sufficiently when it's low on fluid.

There are other reasons to drink plenty of water. Being dehydrated—and an estimated two thirds of people are—diminishes the body's ability to perform virtually every physiological function, including fat metabolism. What's more, when it's low on fluid the body goes in search of water, which results in not just thirst but also a phenomenon that I call "artificial hunger." Although you're not really in need of food, your need for water can make you feel as if you are, leading you to eat when it's not necessary. Another reason you could end up eating more is that dehydration causes the digestive system to work at a diminished capacity, potentially preventing you from getting the nutrients you need and triggering unnecessary eating to make up for the shortfall. On the flip side is the fact that drinking water can actually "drown" your appetite. It's a good bet that if you drink at least six glasses a day, you will have an easier time cutting calories, no matter what diet you're on.

If you're not used to drinking so much water, it may literally seem a little hard to swallow. What may make it easier is remembering that you don't have to drink a lot at once. In fact, it's better to spread out your consumption because drinking more than one to two glasses at one sitting actually stimulates the body to rid itself of water. Always start your morning with a glass of water (that's one down!) and drink one before and after you work out (you're up to three) and one with each meal (that's six—not that hard after all). Carrying a bottle of water with you at all times will also help you reach your quota. Stash one in your car; keep one on your desk and one in your handbag or briefcase. Eventually, I'd like you to work up to nine glasses of water a day, but in the beginning just make sure you get no fewer than six.

When I say "water," I'm referring to plain old water. Not sparkling water, seltzer, or club soda (which has sodium in it) and not vitamin water (which can contain calories). These variations on the theme are fine and even help hydration, but don't figure them into your daily water count.

4. Eliminate alcohol.

To achieve ultimate fitness, I recommend that you eliminate alcohol from your diet for at least these 12 weeks. For some reason, alcohol often doesn't seem to register on many people's calorie radar, although it certainly has a lot of them: at 7 calories per gram, alcohol has more calories than carbohydrates and protein (4 per gram each) and only slightly less than fat (9). It's also absorbed from the stomach into the bloodstream almost immediately, so it doesn't fill you up in the least. When you drink, you're still going to be hungry.

Beyond that, alcohol has properties that will interfere with your goals. For one thing, it's a depressant, which means it slows down everything in the body, including your metabolism (and the effect can linger for days). For another, alcohol, as I'm sure I don't have to tell you, can impair your judgment, including your judgment about how much you should eat.

And there is no question that alcohol impairs your ability to work out in top form. Have a drink or two, and the next day you may feel as though you're trying to exercise with a 10-pound flour sack on your back.

I have nothing against drinking in moderation, particularly now that we know that alcohol—and wine in particular—contains many properties that may help protect against heart disease and cancer. But you are embarking on a 12-week program that's intended to give you striking results in a limited amount of time, and in order for it to succeed you have to make some sacrifices. Alcohol is one of them. While you can certainly put it back into your diet in moderation after the 12 weeks are up, keep it off your menu for now.

5. Make eating a conscious act.

What is a conscious act? Something you do with deliberation and usually by first weighing the potential consequences of your action. When you do something consciously—or mindfully, another word that aptly describes it—you know *what* you're doing and *why.*

This is the kind of thinking I want you to apply to your eating—especially, if emotional eating is a problem for you (as it is for the majority of people who are trying to lose weight). When you eat consciously, you have a far smaller chance of using food for emotional sustenance, and this is particularly important now. I like to think of myself as an optimist, but I'm also a believer in preparing for possible turbulence. During the 12 weeks you spend in this program working hard toward your goal, *something* will inevitably come up. It could be a family crisis, pressure at work, feelings of loneliness or boredom, or just the daily stress of life getting under your skin. If you're an emotional eater and don't have the tools to cope, any of these could potentially knock you off course.

The key to making eating a conscious act lies in self-discovery and inner strength. Much as you did in chapter 1, it's important to ask yourself some tough questions and make some tough decisions. I have rarely seen someone eliminate emotional eating without doing both. It's essential to evaluate what makes you turn to food and how you're going to deal with the problem. And it can be rough. You may have to assess a relationship you're in and whether it can be fixed or needs to be ended. You may have to have an uncomfortable talk with your boss about what's making you unhappy at work. You may need to contemplate changing the kind of work you do or the way you do your current job. Maybe you'll have to seek the help of a financial counselor to assist you in dealing with stressful money issues.

Attacking the source of the problem, which is the only way to end it, is essential. And while the steps you'll need to take to do that can be difficult, once you go after what needs to be changed, you will be a lot closer to getting your life—and as a result, your eating—under control. And—let me just say it again—you should view this as an opportunity. It's a chance to deal with issues that have been swept under the rug and that, when brought out into the open, will help you improve every aspect of your life.

THE CIRCLE OF LIFE

Typically, when I work with a new client who's struggling with emotional eating, I sit down with him or her and ask him or her to take part in an exercise I call the "Circle of Life." The purpose of the exercise is to learn what areas of your life are most important to you—something a lot of people have never asked themselves—then to investigate how things are going in those areas and, if need be, figure out ways to make a change for the better. It's really a process of taking inventory of your life.

It's a very simple exercise: Take a piece of paper and draw a large circle. Next, divide the circle into eight sections, just as you would a pie, one section for each area of your life that is important to you. These categories should be very general, such as career, health, finances, romance, and spirituality. If you can't come up with eight, try to have at least six. Inside each pie piece, write the name of the important aspect of your life. Now look at each section and ask yourself how things are going in that area. If things are going well, write a plus sign in the section; if things aren't going well, write a minus sign.

The minus areas are the ones you want to concentrate on, but don't discount the idea of making the "plus" areas better either.

Write one small thing in each section that you can do today to improve that area of your life, and use that as a road map for the next year. I think you'll be surprised where the map will lead. If you can successfully accomplish one of the small improvements you wrote down each day for a year, your life will be significantly different at the end of that year. If you can do three things a day, *you won't even recognize your life at the end of the year.* It can really be that dramatic—and I've never seen an exception.

When people are successful at getting a grip on their emotional eating, they feel as though a weight has been lifted from their shoulders. Understanding why you are doing something and, through that knowledge, having the power to stop it is enormously freeing. It also generally has a very tangible effect on the body: weight just drops off.

I see becoming a conscious eater as a progression. First, it's important to identify whether or not you are an emotional eater and, if you are, what your triggers are. Your next step is to find a way to regain control over your eating habits. This will take perseverance, but if you learn to cope with life without using food, the rewards will be everlasting.

Sure Signs of (and Reasons for) Emotional Eating

Emotional eaters manifest their problem in lots of different ways. For many people, the classic sign of emotional eating is night eating. Night eaters are often eating in response to anxiety (one reason many people wake up in the middle of the night to eat) or to the emotional turmoil they've experienced throughout the day. Boredom and loneliness are also more likely to come to the surface when the rush of the day is done and the night stretches ahead. If you're an emotional night eater, simply establishing an eating cutoff time for yourself (rule 1) may help you eliminate emotional night eating—though it could also cause your emotional eating to creep into the day, something to be aware of.

Sometimes emotional eating is a reaction to a specific situation. You had a bad day at work. The kids have been so demanding that your nerves are entirely frayed. You and your significant other are fighting. You're helping to care for a friend or family member who's ill and irritable. It doesn't matter what the circumstances are; the end result is that 99 times out of 100 you end up on the couch with a bowl of chips or bag of cookies in your hand, telling yourself it's the only way you can relax.

Other times, people who eat for emotional reasons aren't reacting to any one thing but rather to a life that is in constant turmoil. The cause could be any number of things: dealing with a death or a breakup; feeling depressed about a dead-end job or an unsatisfying relationship. If this sounds familiar, perhaps you even tell yourself that you deserve to eat whatever you want whenever you want because you have it so bad. When things look up, you say to yourself, *then* I'll watch what I eat.

I want to address boredom and loneliness again because they're such common causes of emotional eating, especially loneliness. Food can be a great comfort when you're feeling undervalued or unloved. If there is a void in your life, eating can fill the time and take your mind off the emptiness. But inside you probably know that food can't take the place of love, attention, or engagement in something you find interesting or worthwhile. And what you might not realize is that boredom and loneliness can be two of the most easily remedied causes of emotional eating. Reaching out to other people and finding new things to do can help you virtually eliminate the need to turn to food for company. We'll talk more about this in the next section.

Perhaps you're aware that you're eating out of stress, loneliness, boredom, depression, or any of the many other reasons that cause people to turn to food. In that sense, you are already making eating a conscious act. It's a conscious decision to eat, but your intention—to nurture yourself—won't be realized. And in that sense you're missing the boat. You're conscious of why you're eating but not of the fact that it won't ultimately provide the comfort you need.

On the other hand, you may not be aware of why your eating is out of control, though you have an inkling that it is linked to something you're feeling, something that's perhaps not on the surface but buried deep down inside you. It's absolutely essential, though, that you identify the problem before you can resolve it. Turn again to the truth-telling exercises in chapter 1 to help you. The more soul-searching you do, the better chance you have of becoming someone who makes eating a conscious and deliberate act.

Strategies for Getting a Handle on Emotional Eating

There's no overnight solution to emotional eating. You may think you've conquered it, only to have it raise its ugly head once again during a particularly challenging time. Some people never rid themselves of the temptation to turn to food, and for them it just becomes a matter of managing those impulses. But don't give up; it's important to keep in mind that every emotional eating episode is just one episode. Acknowledge it, think about it, move on. If you feel that you can't overcome the depression or other feelings that are leading you to eat by yourself, you may have to seek the help of a professional therapist. Plenty of people who successfully eliminate emotional eating and make their bodies over take this step, and more often than not it helps tremendously.

There are, though, plenty of things you can do on your own. Each strategy will help bring you more into touch with what you're doing and assist you in finding ways to avoid turning to food for emotional sustenance.

Keep a Journal

Emotional eating is generally a coping tool that develops early in life, and it's often used to help people deal with issues or ways of thinking about themselves that have lingered since childhood. The fact that the behavior is so ingrained is why it's so hard to stop. This is particularly true if you haven't been able to link your eating to any particular stressful event, emotional upheaval, or trauma. But whether you have an inkling of what's behind your behavior or not, I encourage you to use what I think is an invaluable method of self-exploration: keeping a journal.

Keeping a journal, as part of the process of self-discovery, lets you pinpoint why you turn to food for comfort, and that's key to being able to change your behavior. This kind of journal keeping involves keeping track of what you eat, when and where you eat it (i.e., in the middle of the night, standing at the refrigerator), and what you feel at the time. But it's not just a food journal; it's a book that allows you to document your entire day so that you can make the connections between events and your eating. It lets you ask yourself, for instance, "Was I really experiencing physical hunger when I ate?" If you run into an old boyfriend or girlfriend at 10 A.M., feel bad about the way you look (Why couldn't I have looked fabulous so my old flame would rue what he/she was missing?), then by noon are downing a plateful of fish and chips, there's probably a connection. Did the remark your mother made about your weight on the phone annoy you and set you off on a potato chip binge? Chances are you'll get the link if you see it chronicled on the page.

I have a journal available on my Web site www.totalbodymake over.com, that makes recording your day very simple, but you can also create a journal of your own. Begin by carrying your journal with you everywhere so that you can write down everything you ate during an eating episode, what you're feeling, and the events surrounding it while they're fresh in your mind. Then go over what you wrote before bed, adding anything that you might have left out.

The point of keeping a journal is to learn about yourself, then to use that self-knowledge to make adjustments in your life. This is the book on *you*. Use it as a guide to discovering what you didn't know about yourself and changing destructive behavior. You may not see a pattern emerge right away, but eventually relationships between your eating and certain events or feelings will become apparent. Use this knowledge to help you differentiate between real physical hunger and the false tug of emotional hunger. Knowing that you, say, typically head for the vending machines after your boss yells at you can help you realize you need to take a deep breath and get back to work. Are you upset? Yes. Are you truly hungry? No.

Manage Your Meals

Emotional eaters tend to think that anytime they *don't* eat, it's a good thing. But in fact, if you skip meals and let yourself get really hungry in between meals, you will be all the more susceptible to giving in to the tug of eating to satisfy your emotional needs. Make it a point to eat well all day long. Eat a healthy breakfast (rule 1), a moderate lunch, a smallish snack (75 to 150 calories) in between lunch and dinner, and a nutritious, moderate-sized dinner. Note that I used the words "smallish" and "moderate." Stuffing yourself at any one meal can cause your body to secrete an abnormally large amount of insulin, which will encourage your body to store fat. So eat neither too much or too little, and you'll be adding some built-in protection against both emotional eating and weight gain.

Pay Attention While You Eat

For many people, emotional eating is a reward they give themselves. They feel that they are so psychologically black and blue that they deserve some kind of pleasurable consolation prize. But the fact is, you can find pleasure in your meals and snacks if you pay attention to them, and once you do, this may help eliminate your need to eat too much. The trick is to eat consciously. Don't gaze at the TV, drive your car, or stand at the refrigerator as you eat a meal or snack, or you'll never really register the pleasurable aspects of the food. Make eating an event, and make it gratifying.

All too often, especially when eating alone, people shortchange themselves when it comes to food. They don't bother to make or buy anything that resembles a balanced meal and so gyp themselves out of both nutrients and enjoyment. Really make your meals and snacks count. Sit down at the table with someone you can talk to, or if you're alone, even if you're having a frozen dinner or takeout, put it on a plate and eat it with real, not plastic silverware; light a candle, and use an attractive place mat or tablecloth. You'll be surprised at how satisfying regular eating can be if you only pay attention.

Find a Substitute for Food

I love one of the tactics that Tawni (page 12) uses to help her avoid emotional eating: she keeps a pair of athletic shoes in her car so that when she feels upset or stressed out, she can pull over, get out of the car, and take a walk. Exercise is a great substitute for eating, and it's been proven to have a calming effect. Without your even being conscious of it, the workouts you do on this 12-week program should help you cut down on emotional eating—and maybe even eliminate it altogether. But you can be even more deliberate about it. When you feel the urge to eat above and beyond your meals and healthy snacks, head to the gym. Exercise is the perfect substitute for food because it both takes your mind off eating and, in most cases, also suppresses your appetite.

There are also other diversions you can use to keep you from eating. What do you like to do? Read? Talk to friends on the phone? Surf the Internet? Anything that keeps you busy and provides some pleasure can help. Take a class. Take up a craft. Take a walk. Take a bath. Write a letter. Send an e-mail. Learn a foreign language. Do a crossword puzzle. Knit. Garden. Put all those photographs you've been piling up into an album. Reorganize your closet. Choose an activity that will both occupy your mind and improve your mood.

Don't Let Yourself Be Lonely

Food is often used as a substitute for companionship. If that's the trigger for your episodes of emotional eating, get yourself out in the world. Go out and see people whom you like and do things that interest you. Make dates with friends and family, join clubs that focus on your passions, volunteer at a soup kitchen or homeless shelter, sign up for classes in subjects you want to learn more about, visit museums and community offerings, go to parks, and participate in activities such as skating and bowling. Put yourself in the path of other people, and you will be more likely to meet someone with whom you share a special connection. And even if you don't, you'll have an enriching experience. Be a part of life, and life will deliver good things to you.

I know I've said it before, but I think the point can't be made too many times: eliminating emotional eating is a way to change your life. Use this opportunity to discover something about yourself and to make an investment in your future health and happiness.

Making an Investment in Herself
Oprah's Story

I've been in a constant struggle with my weight since I was 22 years old. That's the year that I moved to Baltimore, took a high-profile job as co-anchor of the six o'clock news, and proceeded to gain 10 pounds in less than two weeks.

Apparently I was pretty stressed in my new position, although had you asked me at the time I would have denied it. I was *feeling* no stress or anxiety because I was repressing my real feelings of loneliness and self-doubt. I was on my own for the first time in a city where I knew no one, and there had been a huge ad campaign on every available billboard and bus stop asking, "WHAT IS AN OPRAH?" Talk about pressure to succeed.

But I never really internalized that pressure. I just ate my way through it. Every night after work I'd visit my local mall's food stands, delighting in a baked potato stuffed with bacon and chives and smothered with cheese, followed by a warm, melting chocolate chip cookie. This was my regular routine. It brought me comfort and temporary joy.

When I was wandering the food stalls I never thought about how scary it was to be on my own, how my writing skills hadn't prepared me for the challenge of my new position, or how the entrenched anchorman who I'd been partnered with really felt about having to co-anchor with me. I would stuff myself, then go home to bed.

Using food to repress feelings became a way of life for me. I've eaten my way through good times, great times, sad and challenging events. Strangely enough, I've forgotten major details of many life experiences—like who was actually there and what we did—but I always remember my weight and size. I can look at a tape of any past show, not remember the theme or the guests, but be able to tell you for sure my weight on that date. Unfortunately, my weight and size have had too much power over my life.

Like everyone who has struggled for years and in the end gained more than she or he has lost, I have always wanted to be thin. I wanted to look good in my clothes, to be able to shop for and wear what I liked and not just what fit. I wanted it but wasn't willing to do what it takes to get it or keep it.

I could make all the "most powerful" lists and not feel powerful at all because I had no power over myself. I wanted to be a strong person, but how do you get there when you can't stop eating a bag of chips? An emotional eater. A carbohydrate addict. That was me.

Anyone reading this no doubt has come across a story or two of my oh-so-public dieting woes. I thought I had won the war against weight after connecting with Bob—running a marathon, writing a book about it (*Make the Connection*). After the marathon I kept the weight off, give or take five to eight pounds, for about four years. Then life intervened and I was hit with a one-two punch. I was sued and had to take my show down to Texas during what was an emotionally wrenching trial. I ate pie every night to soothe myself. Around this same time, I poured my heart and soul into the film *Beloved* and it was a box office disappointment. I was devastated. On the morning after the film opened, when I heard that we placed fourth at the box office and would not be on as many screens the next weekend, I asked my chef, Art, to make macaroni and cheese for lunch. I ate my way back up to 208 pounds.

And then one morning my heart literally woke me up. It was racing so fast I thought I could hear it beating. I'd never been aware of my heart beating before, but I could distinctly feel it. I went to the doctor and got an EKG, which was fine. But my blood pressure was 140/87. My doctor told me I needed to lose weight. "Tell me something I don't know," was my first snide thought. I didn't take her advice seriously. I'd been heavier, topping the scale at 237 in the years before I met Bob, and through all that time my blood pressure had remained 110/70.

The palpitations persisted. I went to five different specialists, trying to figure out what was wrong. I went to bed wearing a little black monitor checking my heart rhythms. Nobody could find anything wrong with my heart. But I knew my body was out of balance. I came across the book *The Wisdom of Menopause* and was hit with the unavoidable truth. I was 48 and my hormones were changing. Heart palpitations are a symptom of the change.

Being overweight now wasn't the same as being overweight when I was younger. My heart was resisting the weight and trying every way to let me *feel* it. I got the message. Taking care of yourself and your health is about choosing to live and wanting the best life can offer. You create that offering. I chose to live more healthfully instead of worrying every night if I would awaken in the morning.

I didn't go on an all-out diet, I just started cutting out the white stuff—breads, rice, pasta, my beloved potatoes. I also cut back on salt. My heart stopped racing, my blood pressure dropped. I started sleeping better. My energy level soared. I worked out harder. Ten pounds quickly dropped off. Slowly, just as Bob had predicted, I began losing one to two pounds a week, sometimes even more.

The harder I worked, the better the results, but here is the secret that saved me: not eating after 7:30 PM. Bob had always said to leave at least two hours between bedtime and a meal, which I thought I was doing. But during a period of frustration I said to him, "I'm doing everything right and still holding at 184 pounds for months."

"What are you eating at night?" he asked me.

"I usually have dinner at work," I said, "so I have plenty of time before bed."

"Do you eat when you get home?" Bob asked.

"Not really," I replied.

"What does that mean?"

"I really don't eat a meal. Maybe a handful of nuts, some grapes, a bowl of cereal—all healthy stuff."

Well, Bob pointed out, all of that "healthy stuff" had enough calories to equal a full meal. So I cut out all eating after dinner. Now I don't even have a grape past 7:30 PM. I dropped another eight pounds within a month.

I had done some weight training before, but now I got serious about it. I like the way it makes me feel strong and in control. Weight training also curtails two of the most dramatic effects of aging: decreased bone density and muscle mass. Here's my new routine now: a minimum of 30 minutes aerobic exercise, six days a week; I also strength-train every other day. I still avoid the white stuff—breads, refined sugars, pastas—except for on Christmas and my birthday and two other special occasions during the year. And, again, I don't consume a morsel after 7:30 PM. This works for me. I'm in better shape now than I've ever been. Stronger, more flexible. No heart palpitations. I feel so alive; like my life is blazing at a thousand degrees. I've come a long way since wandering the food stalls at the mall.

What I know for sure is that there is no shortcut to weight loss. It's an investment you make in yourself every day. I finally get it. I choose to live!

4

THE 12-WEEK TOTAL BODY MAKEOVER PLAN

YOU'RE ABOUT TO MAKE a great investment in yourself. Over the next twelve weeks, the Total Body Makeover will give you an opportunity to go beyond pushing your physical limits and try your psychological mettle as well; every day will be a test of your commitment, your dedication, your inner strength, and your strength of character. When you succeed here, you will walk away knowing that you possess qualities that will help you be successful in anything you do in life.

Following the Plan

All the exercise you need to do is outlined in the following week-by-week charts. Combined with the five simple eating rules covered in the preceding chapter, it will help you change not just your body, but your life.

Now a bit about the charts. All the functional and strength-training exercises are numbered so that you can correlate them to the exercise photos and instructions in chapter 2. Do you have to follow them in numerical order? No. You can do them in whatever order you like, especially the stretches. That said, what you might let guide you in determining the order of the strength-training exercises is which muscles you're going to be working. There is a slight advantage to working your larger muscle groups first, since that will help your body warm up more quickly. In that case, you'd do the leg exercises first and arm and shoulder exercises last. But don't be tied to that order, especially at the gym, when there might be somebody else using the machine that's next on your list. Better to keep going than to wait.

On some days you'll be doing functional exercises, strength-training exercises, and aerobic exercises all in one session. I'm often asked if it's better to do the strength-training part or the aerobic exercise part first. Personally, I prefer doing weights first since it allows me to ease into working out a little more leisurely. I'd also rather not do weights when I'm all sweaty and have to worry about mopping up after myself at each station (I highly recommend being considerate of the next exerciser!). Also, most gyms have the air-conditioning on, which I don't like when I'm hot and perspiring. Some people, however, swear there's magic in doing cardiovascular exercise before weights. Again, this one's up to you.

If you're going to break up your workouts into A.M. and P.M. sessions, I recommend that you do the aerobic exercise in the morning. That way you'll get its metabolism-revving benefit all day long. A morning aerobic workout may also help dull your appetite so that you consume fewer calories as the day goes along. While we're on the subject of aerobic exercise, I want to note that the 2-minute increase in duration that I propose for each week is just a guideline. If you're training for a race or other event, you may want to add more time. Likewise, if the extra two minutes is outside of your ability in any given week, adjust the time accordingly.

Exactly when you work out is less important than adhering consistently to the program. Devote the next 12 weeks to this program by making it your top priority, and I promise you that you'll change your body—and quite possibly your life!

WEEK 1
FUNCTIONAL EXERCISES (PP. 88–102)

EXERCISE	BEGINNER WEEKLY GOAL	INTERMEDIATE WEEKLY GOAL	ADVANCED WEEKLY GOAL
1. Hamstring Stretch	2–3 stretches, 6 times a week	3 stretches, 6 times a week	3 stretches, 6 times a week
2. Quadriceps Stretch	2–3 stretches, 6 times a week	3 stretches, 6 times a week	3 stretches, 6 times a week
3. Upper Calf Stretch	2–3 stretches, 6 times a week	3 stretches, 6 times a week	3 stretches, 6 times a week
4. Lower Calf Stretch	2–3 stretches, 6 times a week	3 stretches, 6 times a week	3 stretches, 6 times a week
5. Middle and Lower Back Stretch	2–3 stretches, 6 times a week	3 stretches, 6 times a week	3 stretches, 6 times a week
6. Basic Crunches	1–2 sets, 6 times a week	3 sets, 6 times a week	3 sets; do either this exercise or Incline Sit-Ups 6 times a week, alternating between the two
7. Twisting Trunk Curl Crunches	1–2 sets, 6 times a week	3 sets, 6 times a week	3 sets, 6 times a week

Exercise			
8. Upper Abdomen Crunches	1–2 sets, 6 times a week	3 sets, 6 times a week	3 sets, 6 times a week
9. Arm and Leg Raise	1–2 sets, 6 times a week	3 sets, 6 times a week	3 sets, 6 times a week
10. Shrug Roll	1–2 sets, 6 times a week	3 sets, 6 times a week	3 sets, 6 times a week
11. Heel Raises	1–2 sets, 6 times a week	3 sets, 6 times a week	3 sets, 6 times a week
12. Reverse Trunk Curl			3 sets, 6 times a week
13. Extended Arm Crunch			3 sets, 6 times a week
14. Vertical Leg Crunch			3 sets, 6 times a week
15. Incline Sit-Up			3 sets; do either this exercise or Basic Crunches 6 times a week, alternating between the two

STRENGTH-TRAINING EXERCISES (PP. 123–141)

EXERCISES	BEGINNER WEEKLY GOAL	INTERMEDIATE WEEKLY GOAL	ADVANCED WEEKLY GOAL
1. Squats	1–2 sets, 3 times a week	3 sets, 3 times a week	3 sets, every other day
2. Lunges	1–2 sets, 3 times a week	3 sets, 3 times a week	3 sets, every other day
3. Chest Press	1–2 sets, 3 times a week	3 sets, 3 times a week	3 sets, every other day
4. Shoulder Press	1–2 sets, 3 times a week	3 sets, 3 times a week	3 sets, every other day
5. Butterfly	1–2 sets, 3 times a week	3 sets, 3 times a week	3 sets, every other day
6. Dumbbell Fly	1–2 sets, 3 times a week	3 sets, 3 times a week	3 sets, every other day
7. Biceps Curl	1–2 sets, 3 times a week	3 sets, 3 times a week	3 sets, every other day
8. Triceps Extension	1–2 sets, 3 times a week	3 sets, 3 times a week	3 sets, every other day
9. One-Arm Row		3 sets, 3 times a week	3 sets, every other day
10. Lateral Raise		3 sets, 3 times a week	3 sets, every other day
11. Leg Press		3 sets, 3 times a week	3 sets, every other day
12. Leg Extension		3 sets, 3 times a week	3 sets, every other day

13. Leg Curl		3 sets, 3 times a week	3 sets, every other day
14. Incline Press			3 sets, every other day
15. Upright Row			3 sets, every other day

AEROBIC EXERCISE (PP. 114–117)

AEROBIC WORKOUT	BEGINNER WEEKLY GOAL	INTERMEDIATE WEEKLY GOAL	ADVANCED WEEKLY GOAL
Regular Workout (your choice) at a 7–8 intensity	15 minutes or as much as you can do, 5 days a week	30 minutes, 5 days a week	45 minutes, 5 days a week
Double Workout (your choice) at a 6–7 intensity	30 minutes or as much as you can do, 1 day a week	60 minutes, 1 day a week	90 minutes, 1 day a week

WEEK 2
FUNCTIONAL EXERCISES (PP. 88–102)

EXERCISES WEEKLY GOAL	BEGINNER WEEKLY GOAL	INTERMEDIATE WEEKLY GOAL	ADVANCED WEEKLY GOAL
1. Hamstring Stretch	2–3 stretches, 6 times a week	3 stretches, 6 times a week	3 stretches, 6 times a week
2. Quadriceps Stretch	2–3 stretches, 6 times a week	3 stretches, 6 times a week	3 stretches, 6 times a week
3. Upper Calf Stretch	2–3 stretches, 6 times a week	3 stretches, 6 times a week	3 stretches, 6 times a week
4. Lower Calf Stretch	2–3 stretches, 6 times a week	3 stretches, 6 times a week	3 stretches, 6 times a week
5. Middle and Lower Back Stretch	2–3 stretches, 6 times a week	3 stretches, 6 times a week	3 stretches, 6 times a week
6. Basic Crunches	1–2 sets, 6 times a week	3 sets, 6 times a week	3 sets; do either this exercise or Incline Sit-Up 6 times a week, alternating between the two
7. Twisting Trunk Curl Crunches	1–2 sets, 6 times a week	3 sets, 6 times a week	3 sets, 6 times a week

Exercise			
8. Upper Abdomen Crunches	1–2 sets, 6 times a week	3 sets, 6 times a week	3 sets, 6 times a week
9. Arm and Leg Raise	1–2 sets, 6 times a week	3 sets, 6 times a week	3 sets, 6 times a week
10. Shrug Roll	1–2 sets, 6 times a week	3 sets, 6 times a week	3 sets, 6 times a week
11. Heel Raises	1–2 sets, 6 times a week	3 sets, 6 times a week	3 sets, 6 times a week
12. Reverse Trunk Curl			3 sets, 6 times a week
13. Extended Arm Crunch			3 sets, 6 times a week
14. Vertical Leg Crunch			3 sets, 6 times a week
15. Incline Sit-Up			3 sets; do either this exercise or Basic Crunches 6 times a week, alternating between the two

STRENGTH-TRAINING EXERCISES (PP. 123–141)

EXERCISES	BEGINNER WEEKLY GOAL	INTERMEDIATE WEEKLY GOAL	ADVANCED WEEKLY GOAL
1. Squats	1–2 sets, 3 times a week	3 sets, 3 times a week	3 sets, every other day
2. Lunges	1–2 sets, 3 times a week	3 sets, 3 times a week	3 sets, every other day
3. Chest Press	1–2 sets, 3 times a week	3 sets, 3 times a week	3 sets, every other day
4. Shoulder Press	1–2 sets, 3 times a week	3 sets, 3 times a week	3 sets, every other day
5. Butterfly	1–2 sets, 3 times a week	3 sets, 3 times a week	3 sets, every other day
6. Dumbbell Fly	1–2 sets, 3 times a week	3 sets, 3 times a week	3 sets, every other day
7. Biceps Curl	1–2 sets, 3 times a week	3 sets, 3 times a week	3 sets, every other day
8. Triceps Extension	1–2 sets, 3 times a week	3 sets, 3 times a week	3 sets, every other day
9. One-Arm Row		3 sets, 3 times a week	3 sets, every other day
10. Lateral Raise		3 sets, 3 times a week	3 sets, every other day
11. Leg Press		3 sets, 3 times a week	3 sets, every other day
12. Leg Extension		3 sets, 3 times a week	3 sets, every other day

	INTERMEDIATE	ADVANCED
13. Leg Curl	3 sets, 3 times a week	3 sets, every other day
14. Incline Press		3 sets, every other day
15. Upright Row		3 sets, every other day

AEROBIC EXERCISE (PP. 114–117)

AEROBIC WORKOUT	BEGINNER WEEKLY GOAL	INTERMEDIATE WEEKLY GOAL	ADVANCED WEEKLY GOAL
Regular Workout (your choice) at a 7–8 intensity	17 minutes or as much as you can do, 5 days a week	32 minutes, 5 days a week	47 minutes, 5 days a week
Double Workout (your choice) at a 6–7 intensity	34 minutes or as much as you can do, 1 day a week	64 minutes, 1 day a week	94 minutes, 1 day a week

WEEK 3
FUNCTIONAL EXERCISES (PP. 88–102)

EXERCISES	BEGINNER WEEKLY GOAL	INTERMEDIATE WEEKLY GOAL	ADVANCED WEEKLY GOAL
1. Hamstring Stretch	2–3 stretches, 6 times a week	3 stretches, 6 times a week	3 stretches, 6 times a week
2. Quadriceps Stretch	2–3 stretches, 6 times a week	3 stretches, 6 times a week	3 stretches, 6 times a week
3. Upper Calf Stretch	2–3 stretches, 6 times a week	3 stretches, 6 times a week	3 stretches, 6 times a week
4. Lower Calf Stretch	2–3 stretches, 6 times a week	3 stretches, 6 times a week	3 stretches, 6 times a week
5. Middle and Lower Back Stretch	2–3 stretches, 6 times a week	3 stretches, 6 times a week	3 stretches, 6 times a week
6. Basic Crunches	1–2 sets, 6 times a week	3 sets, 6 times a week	3 sets; do either this exercise or Incline Sit-Up 6 times a week, alternating between the two
7. Twisting Trunk Curl Crunches	1–2 sets, 6 times a week	3 sets, 6 times a week	3 sets, 6 times a week

8. Upper Abdomen Crunches	1–2 sets, 6 times a week	3 sets, 6 times a week	3 sets, 6 times a week
9. Arm and Leg Raise	1–2 sets, 6 times a week	3 sets, 6 times a week	3 sets, 6 times a week
10. Shrug Roll	1–2 sets, 6 times a week	3 sets, 6 times a week	3 sets, 6 times a week
11. Heel Raises	1–2 sets, 6 times a week	3 sets, 6 times a week	3 sets, 6 times a week
12. Reverse Trunk Curl			3 sets, 6 times a week
13. Extended Arm Crunch			3 sets, 6 times a week
14. Vertical Leg Crunch			3 sets, 6 times a week
15. Incline Sit-Up			3 sets; do either this exercise or Basic Crunches 6 times a week, alternating between the two

STRENGTH-TRAINING EXERCISES (PP. 123–141)

EXERCISES	BEGINNER WEEKLY GOAL	INTERMEDIATE WEEKLY GOAL	ADVANCED WEEKLY GOAL
1. Squats	1–2 sets, 3 times a week	3 sets, 3 times a week	3 sets, every other day
2. Lunges	1–2 sets, 3 times a week	3 sets, 3 times a week	3 sets, every other day
3. Chest Press	1–2 sets, 3 times a week	3 sets, 3 times a week	3 sets, every other day
4. Shoulder Press	1–2 sets, 3 times a week	3 sets, 3 times a week	3 sets, every other day
5. Butterfly	1–2 sets, 3 times a week	3 sets, 3 times a week	3 sets, every other day
6. Dumbbell Fly	1–2 sets, 3 times a week	3 sets, 3 times a week	3 sets, every other day
7. Biceps Curl	1–2 sets, 3 times a week	3 sets, 3 times a week	3 sets, every other day
8. Triceps Extension	1–2 sets, 3 times a week	3 sets, 3 times a week	3 sets, every other day
9. One-Arm Row		3 sets, 3 times a week	3 sets, every other day
10. Lateral Raise		3 sets, 3 times a week	3 sets, every other day
11. Leg Press		3 sets, 3 times a week	3 sets, every other day
12. Leg Extension		3 sets, 3 times a week	3 sets, every other day

13. Leg Curl	3 sets, 3 times a week		3 sets, every other day
14. Incline Press			3 sets, every other day
15. Upright Row			3 sets, every other day

AEROBIC EXERCISE (PP. 114–117)

AEROBIC WORKOUT	BEGINNER WEEKLY GOAL	INTERMEDIATE WEEKLY GOAL	ADVANCED WEEKLY GOAL
Regular Workout (your choice) at a 7–8 intensity	19 minutes or as much as you can do, 5 days a week	34 minutes, 5 days a week	49 minutes, 5 days a week
Double Workout (your choice) at a 6–7 intensity	38 minutes or as much as you can do, 1 day a week	68 minutes, 1 day a week	98 minutes, 1 day a week

WEEK 4
FUNCTIONAL EXERCISES (PP. 88–102)

EXERCISES	BEGINNER WEEKLY GOAL	INTERMEDIATE WEEKLY GOAL	ADVANCED WEEKLY GOAL
1. Hamstring Stretch	2–3 stretches, 6 times a week	3 stretches, 6 times a week	3 stretches, 6 times a week
2. Quadriceps Stretch	2–3 stretches, 6 times a week	3 stretches, 6 times a week	3 stretches, 6 times a week
3. Upper Calf Stretch	2–3 stretches, 6 times a week	3 stretches, 6 times a week	3 stretches, 6 times a week
4. Lower Calf Stretch	2–3 stretches, 6 times a week	3 stretches, 6 times a week	3 stretches, 6 times a week
5. Middle and Lower Back Stretch	2–3 stretches, 6 times a week	3 stretches, 6 times a week	3 stretches, 6 times a week
6. Basic Crunches	1–2 sets, 6 times a week	3 sets, 6 times a week	3 sets; do either this exercise or Incline Sit-Up 6 times a week, alternating between the two
7. Twisting Trunk Curl Crunches	1–2 sets, 6 times a week	3 sets, 6 times a week	3 sets, 6 times a week

Exercise			
8. Upper Abdomen Crunches	1–2 sets, 6 times a week	3 sets, 6 times a week	3 sets, 6 times a week
9. Arm and Leg Raise	1–2 sets, 6 times a week	3 sets, 6 times a week	3 sets, 6 times a week
10. Shrug Roll	1–2 sets, 6 times a week	3 sets, 6 times a week	3 sets, 6 times a week
11. Heel Raises	1–2 sets, 6 times a week	3 sets, 6 times a week	3 sets, 6 times a week
12. Reverse Trunk Curl			3 sets, 6 times a week
13. Extended Arm Crunch			3 sets, 6 times a week
14. Vertical Leg Crunch			3 sets, 6 times a week
15. Incline Sit-Up			3 sets; do either this exercise or Basic Crunches 6 times a week, alternating between the two

STRENGTH-TRAINING EXERCISES (PP. 123–141)

EXERCISES	BEGINNER WEEKLY GOAL	INTERMEDIATE WEEKLY GOAL	ADVANCED WEEKLY GOAL
1. Squats	1–2 sets, 3 times a week	3 sets, 3 times a week	3 sets, every other day
2. Lunges	1–2 sets, 3 times a week	3 sets, 3 times a week	3 sets, every other day
3. Chest Press	1–2 sets, 3 times a week	3 sets, 3 times a week	3 sets, every other day
4. Shoulder Press	1–2 sets, 3 times a week	3 sets, 3 times a week	3 sets, every other day
5. Butterfly	1–2 sets, 3 times a week	3 sets, 3 times a week	3 sets, every other day
6. Dumbbell Fly	1–2 sets, 3 times a week	3 sets, 3 times a week	3 sets, every other day
7. Biceps Curl	1–2 sets, 3 times a week	3 sets, 3 times a week	3 sets, every other day
8. Triceps Extension	1–2 sets, 3 times a week	3 sets, 3 times a week	3 sets, every other day
9. One-Arm Row		3 sets, 3 times a week	3 sets, every other day
10. Lateral Raise		3 sets, 3 times a week	3 sets, every other day
11. Leg Press		3 sets, 3 times a week	3 sets, every other day
12. Leg Extension		3 sets, 3 times a week	3 sets, every other day

13. Leg Curl	3 sets, 3 times a week		3 sets, every other day
14. Incline Press			3 sets, every other day
15. Upright Row			3 sets, every other day

AEROBIC EXERCISE (PP. 114–117)

AEROBIC WORKOUT	BEGINNER WEEKLY GOAL	INTERMEDIATE WEEKLY GOAL	ADVANCED WEEKLY GOAL
Regular Workout (your choice) at a 7–8 intensity	21 minutes or as much as you can do, 5 days a week	36 minutes, 5 days a week	51 minutes, 5 days a week
Double Workout (your choice) at a 6–7 intensity	42 minutes or as much as you can do, 1 day a week	72 minutes, 1 day a week	102 minutes, 1 day a week

WEEK 5
FUNCTIONAL EXERCISES (PP. 88–102)

EXERCISES	BEGINNER WEEKLY GOAL	INTERMEDIATE WEEKLY GOAL	ADVANCED WEEKLY GOAL
1. Hamstring Stretch	2–3 stretches, 6 times a week	3 stretches, 6 times a week	3 stretches, 6 times a week
2. Quadriceps Stretch	2–3 stretches, 6 times a week	3 stretches, 6 times a week	3 stretches, 6 times a week
3. Upper Calf Stretch	2–3 stretches, 6 times a week	3 stretches, 6 times a week	3 stretches, 6 times a week
4. Lower Calf Stretch	2–3 stretches, 6 times a week	3 stretches, 6 times a week	3 stretches, 6 times a week
5. Middle and Lower Back Stretch	2–3 stretches, 6 times a week	3 stretches, 6 times a week	3 stretches, 6 times a week
6. Basic Crunches	1–2 sets, 6 times a week	3 sets, 6 times a week	3 sets, do either this exercise or Incline Sit-Up 6 times a week alternating between the two
7. Twisting Trunk Curl Crunches	1–2 sets, 6 times a week	3 sets, 6 times a week	3 sets, 6 times a week

8. Upper Abdomen Crunches	1–2 sets, 6 times a week	3 sets, 6 times a week	3 sets, 6 times a week
9. Arm and Leg Raise	1–2 sets, 6 times a week	3 sets, 6 times a week	3 sets, 6 times a week
10. Shrug Roll	1–2 sets, 6 times a week	3 sets, 6 times a week	3 sets, 6 times a week
11. Heel Raises	1–2 sets, 6 times a week	3 sets, 6 times a week	3 sets, 6 times a week
12. Reverse Trunk Curl			3 sets, 6 times a week
13. Extended Arm Crunch			3 sets, 6 times a week
14. Vertical Leg Crunch			3 sets, 6 times a week
15. Incline Sit-Up			3 sets; do either this exercise or Basic Crunches 6 times a week, alternating between the two

STRENGTH-TRAINING EXERCISES (PP. 123–141)

EXERCISES	BEGINNER WEEKLY GOAL	INTERMEDIATE WEEKLY GOAL	ADVANCED WEEKLY GOAL
1. Squats	1–2 sets, 3 times a week	3 sets, 3 times a week	3 sets, every other day
2. Lunges	1–2 sets, 3 times a week	3 sets, 3 times a week	3 sets, every other day
3. Chest Press	1–2 sets, 3 times a week	3 sets, 3 times a week	3 sets, every other day
4. Shoulder Press	1–2 sets, 3 times a week	3 sets, 3 times a week	3 sets, every other day
5. Butterfly	1–2 sets, 3 times a week	3 sets, 3 times a week	3 sets, every other day
6. Dumbbell Fly	1–2 sets, 3 times a week	3 sets, 3 times a week	3 sets, every other day
7. Biceps Curl	1–2 sets, 3 times a week	3 sets, 3 times a week	3 sets, every other day
8. Triceps Extension	1–2 sets, 3 times a week	3 sets, 3 times a week	3 sets, every other day
9. One-Arm Row		3 sets, 3 times a week	3 sets, every other day
10. Lateral Raise		3 sets, 3 times a week	3 sets, every other day
11. Leg Press		3 sets, 3 times a week	3 sets, every other day
12. Leg Extension		3 sets, 3 times a week	3 sets, every other day

13. Leg Curl	3 sets, 3 times a week	3 sets, every other day
14. Incline Press		3 sets, every other day
15. Upright Row		3 sets, every other day

AEROBIC EXERCISE (PP. 114–117)

AEROBIC WORKOUT	BEGINNER WEEKLY GOAL	INTERMEDIATE WEEKLY GOAL	ADVANCED WEEKLY GOAL
Regular Workout (your choice) at a 7–8 intensity	23 minutes or as much as you can do, 5 days a week	38 minutes, 5 days a week	53 minutes, 5 days a week
Double Workout (your choice) at a 6–7 intensity	46 minutes or as much as you can do, 1 day a week	76 minutes, 1 day a week	106 minutes, 1 day a week

WEEK 6
FUNCTIONAL EXERCISES (PP. 88–102)

EXERCISES	BEGINNER WEEKLY GOAL	INTERMEDIATE WEEKLY GOAL	ADVANCED WEEKLY GOAL
1. Hamstring Stretch	2–3 stretches, 6 times a week	3 stretches, 6 times a week	3 stretches, 6 times a week
2. Quadriceps Stretch	2–3 stretches, 6 times a week	3 stretches, 6 times a week	3 stretches, 6 times a week
3. Upper Calf Stretch	2–3 stretches, 6 times a week	3 stretches, 6 times a week	3 stretches, 6 times a week
4. Lower Calf Stretch	2–3 stretches, 6 times a week	3 stretches, 6 times a week	3 stretches, 6 times a week
5. Middle and Lower Back Stretch	2–3 stretches, 6 times a week	3 stretches, 6 times a week	3 stretches, 6 times a week
6. Basic Crunches	1–2 sets, 6 times a week	3 sets, 6 times a week	3 sets; do either this exercise or Incline Sit-Up 6 times a week, alternating between the two

Exercise			
7. Twisting Trunk Curl Crunches	1–2 sets, 6 times a week	3 sets, 6 times a week	3 sets, 6 times a week
8. Upper Abdomen Crunches	1–2 sets, 6 times a week	3 sets, 6 times a week	3 sets, 6 times a week
9. Arm and Leg Raise	1–2 sets, 6 times a week	3 sets, 6 times a week	3 sets, 6 times a week
10. Shrug Roll	1–2 sets, 6 times a week	3 sets, 6 times a week	3 sets, 6 times a week
11. Heel Raises	1–2 sets, 6 times a week	3 sets, 6 times a week	3 sets, 6 times a week
12. Reverse Trunk Curl			3 sets, 6 times a week
13. Extended Arm Crunch			3 sets, 6 times a week
14. Vertical Leg Crunch			3 sets, 6 times a week
15. Incline Sit-Up			3 sets; do either this exercise or Basic Crunches 6 times a week, alternating between the two

STRENGTH-TRAINING EXERCISES (PP. 123–141)

EXERCISES	BEGINNER WEEKLY GOAL	INTERMEDIATE WEEKLY GOAL	ADVANCED WEEKLY GOAL
1. Squats	1–2 sets, 3 times a week	3 sets, 3 times a week	3 sets, every other day
2. Lunges	1–2 sets, 3 times a week	3 sets, 3 times a week	3 sets, every other day
3. Chest Press	1–2 sets, 3 times a week	3 sets, 3 times a week	3 sets, every other day
4. Shoulder Press	1–2 sets, 3 times a week	3 sets, 3 times a week	3 sets, every other day
5. Butterfly	1–2 sets, 3 times a week	3 sets, 3 times a week	3 sets, every other day
6. Dumbbell Fly	1–2 sets, 3 times a week	3 sets, 3 times a week	3 sets, every other day
7. Biceps Curl	1–2 sets, 3 times a week	3 sets, 3 times a week	3 sets, every other day
8. Triceps Extension	1–2 sets, 3 times a week	3 sets, 3 times a week	3 sets, every other day
9. One-Arm Row		3 sets, 3 times a week	3 sets, every other day
10. Lateral Raise		3 sets, 3 times a week	3 sets, every other day
11. Leg Press		3 sets, 3 times a week	3 sets, every other day
12. Leg Extension		3 sets, 3 times a week	3 sets, every other day

13. Leg Curl	3 sets, 3 times a week	3 sets, every other day
14. Upright Row		3 sets, every other day
15. Incline Press	3 sets, 3 times a week	3 sets, every other day

AEROBIC EXERCISE (PP. 114–117)

AEROBIC WORKOUT	BEGINNER WEEKLY GOAL	INTERMEDIATE WEEKLY GOAL	ADVANCED WEEKLY GOAL
Regular Workout (your choice) at a 7–8 intensity	25 minutes or as much as you can do, 5 days a week	40 minutes, 5 days a week	55 minutes, 5 days a week
Double Workout (your choice) at a 6–7 intensity	50 minutes or as much as you can do, 1 day a week	80 minutes, 1 day a week	110 minutes, 1 day a week

WEEK 7
FUNCTIONAL EXERCISES (PP. 88–102)

EXERCISES	BEGINNER WEEKLY GOAL	INTERMEDIATE WEEKLY GOAL	ADVANCED WEEKLY GOAL
1. Hamstring Stretch	2–3 stretches, 6 times a week	3 stretches, 6 times a week	3 stretches, 6 times a week
2. Quadriceps Stretch	2–3 stretches, 6 times a week	3 stretches, 6 times a week	3 stretches, 6 times a week
3. Upper Calf Stretch	2–3 stretches, 6 times a week	3 stretches, 6 times a week	3 stretches, 6 times a week
4. Lower Calf Stretch	2–3 stretches, 6 times a week	3 stretches, 6 times a week	3 stretches, 6 times a week
5. Middle and Lower Back Stretch	2–3 stretches, 6 times a week	3 stretches, 6 times a week	3 stretches, 6 times a week
6. Basic Crunches	2–3 sets, 6 times a week	3 sets, 6 times a week	3 sets; do either this exercise or Incline Sit-Up 6 times a week, alternating between the two

7. Twisting Trunk Curl Crunches	2–3 sets, 6 times a week	3 sets, 6 times a week	3 sets, 6 times a week
8. Upper Abdomen Crunches	2–3 sets, 6 times a week	3 sets, 6 times a week	3 sets, 6 times a week
9. Arm and Leg Raise	2–3 sets, 6 times a week	3 sets, 6 times a week	3 sets, 6 times a week
10. Shrug Roll	2–3 sets, 6 times a week	3 sets, 6 times a week	3 sets, 6 times a week
11. Heel Raises	2–3 sets, 6 times a week	3 sets, 6 times a week	3 sets, 6 times a week
12. Reverse Trunk Curl			3 sets, 6 times a week
13. Extended Arm Crunch			3 sets, 6 times a week
14. Vertical Leg Crunch			3 sets, 6 times a week
15. Incline Sit-Up			3 sets; do either this exercise or Basic Crunches 6 times a week, alternating between the two

STRENGTH-TRAINING EXERCISES (PP. 123–141)

EXERCISES	BEGINNER WEEKLY GOAL	INTERMEDIATE WEEKLY GOAL	ADVANCED WEEKLY GOAL
1. Squats	2–3 sets, 3 times a week	3 sets, every other day	3 sets, every other day
2. Lunges	2–3 sets, 3 times a week	3 sets, every other day	3 sets, every other day
3. Chest Press	2–3 sets, 3 times a week	3 sets, every other day	3 sets, every other day
4. Shoulder Press	2–3 sets, 3 times a week	3 sets, every other day	3 sets, every other day
5. Butterfly	2–3 sets, 3 times a week	3 sets, every other day	3 sets, every other day
6. Dumbbell Fly	2–3 sets, 3 times a week	3 sets, every other day	3 sets, every other day
7. Biceps Curl	2–3 sets, 3 times a week	3 sets, every other day	3 sets, every other day
8. Triceps Extension	2–3 sets, 3 times a week	3 sets, every other day	3 sets, every other day
9. One-Arm Row	2–3 sets, 3 times a week	3 sets, every other day	3 sets, every other day
10. Lateral Raise	2–3 sets, 3 times a week	3 sets, every other day	3 sets, every other day
11. Leg Press		3 sets, every other day	3 sets, every other day
12. Leg Extension		3 sets, every other day	3 sets, every other day
13. Leg Curl		3 sets, every other day	3 sets, every other day

	INTERMEDIATE	ADVANCED
14. Incline Press	3 sets, every other day	3 sets, every other day
15. Upright Row	3 sets, every other day	3 sets, every other day
16. Thumbs Down		3 sets, every other day
17. Frontal Raise		3 sets, every other day
18. External Rotation		3 sets, every other day
19. Lat Pull-Down		3 sets, every other day

AEROBIC EXERCISE (PP. 114–117)

AEROBIC WORKOUT	BEGINNER WEEKLY GOAL	INTERMEDIATE WEEKLY GOAL	ADVANCED WEEKLY GOAL
Regular Workout (your choice) at a 7–8 intensity	27 minutes or as much as you can do, 5 days a week	42 minutes, 5 days a week	57 minutes, 5 days a week
Double Workout (your choice) at a 6–7 intensity	54 minutes or as much as you can do, 1 day a week	84 minutes, 1 day a week	114 minutes, 1 day a week

WEEK 8
FUNCTIONAL EXERCISES (PP. 88–102)

EXERCISES	BEGINNER WEEKLY GOAL	INTERMEDIATE WEEKLY GOAL	ADVANCED WEEKLY GOAL
1. Hamstring Stretch	2–3 stretches, 6 times a week	3 stretches, 6 times a week	3 stretches, 6 times a week
2. Quadriceps Stretch	2–3 stretches, 6 times a week	3 stretches, 6 times a week	3 stretches, 6 times a week
3. Upper Calf Stretch	2–3 stretches, 6 times a week	3 stretches, 6 times a week	3 stretches, 6 times a week
4. Lower Calf Stretch	2–3 stretches, 6 times a week	3 stretches, 6 times a week	3 stretches, 6 times a week
5. Middle and Lower Back Stretch	2–3 stretches, 6 times a week	3 stretches, 6 times a week	3 stretches, 6 times a week
6. Basic Crunches	2–3 sets, 6 times a week	3 sets, 6 times a week	3 sets, do either this exercise or Incline Sit-Up 6 times a week, alternating between the two
7. Twisting Trunk Curl Crunches	2–3 sets, 6 times a week	3 sets, 6 times a week	3 sets, 6 times a week

Exercise			
8. Upper Abdomen Crunches	2–3 sets, 6 times a week	3 sets, 6 times a week	3 sets, 6 times a week
9. Arm and Leg Raise	2–3 sets, 6 times a week	3 sets, 6 times a week	3 sets, 6 times a week
10. Shrug Roll	2–3 sets, 6 times a week	3 sets, 6 times a week	3 sets, 6 times a week
11. Heel Raises	2–3 sets, 6 times a week	3 sets, 6 times a week	3 sets, 6 times a week
12. Reverse Trunk Curl			3 sets, 6 times a week
13. Extended Arm Crunch			3 sets, 6 times a week
14. Vertical Leg Crunch			3 sets, 6 times a week
15. Incline Sit-Up			3 sets; do either this exercise or Basic Crunches 6 times a week, alternating between the two

STRENGTH-TRAINING EXERCISES (PP. 123–141)

EXERCISES	BEGINNER WEEKLY GOAL	INTERMEDIATE WEEKLY GOAL	ADVANCED WEEKLY GOAL
1. Squats	2–3 sets, 3 times a week	3 sets, every other day	3 sets, every other day
2. Lunges	2–3 sets, 3 times a week	3 sets, every other day	3 sets, every other day
3. Chest Press	2–3 sets, 3 times a week	3 sets, every other day	3 sets, every other day
4. Shoulder Press	2–3 sets, 3 times a week	3 sets, every other day	3 sets, every other day
5. Butterfly	2–3 sets, 3 times a week	3 sets, every other day	3 sets, every other day
6. Dumbbell Fly	2–3 sets, 3 times a week	3 sets, every other day	3 sets, every other day
7. Biceps Curl	2–3 sets, 3 times a week	3 sets, every other day	3 sets, every other day
8. Triceps Extension	2–3 sets, 3 times a week	3 sets, every other day	3 sets, every other day
9. One-Arm Row	2–3 sets, 3 times a week	3 sets, every other day	3 sets, every other day
10. Lateral Raise	2–3 sets, 3 times a week	3 sets, every other day	3 sets, every other day
11. Leg Press		3 sets, every other day	3 sets, every other day
12. Leg Extension		3 sets, every other day	3 sets, every other day
13. Leg Curl		3 sets, every other day	3 sets, every other day

Exercise		
14. Upright Row		3 sets, every other day
15. Incline Press	3 sets, every other day	3 sets, every other day
16. Thumbs Down		3 sets, every other day
17. Frontal Raise		3 sets, every other day
18. External Rotation		3 sets, every other day
19. Lat Pull-Down	3 sets, every other day	3 sets, every other day

AEROBIC EXERCISE (PP. 114–117)

AEROBIC WORKOUT	BEGINNER WEEKLY GOAL	INTERMEDIATE WEEKLY GOAL	ADVANCED WEEKLY GOAL
Regular Workout (your choice) at a 7–8 intensity	29 minutes or as much as you can do, 5 days a week	44 minutes, 5 days a week	59 minutes, 5 days a week
Double Workout (your choice) at a 6–7 intensity	58 minutes or as much as you can do, 1 day a week	88 minutes, 1 day a week	118 minutes, 1 day a week

WEEK 9
FUNCTIONAL EXERCISES (PP. 88–102)

EXERCISES	BEGINNER WEEKLY GOAL	INTERMEDIATE WEEKLY GOAL	ADVANCED WEEKLY GOAL
1. Hamstring Stretch	2–3 stretches, 6 times a week	3 stretches, 6 times a week	3 stretches, 6 times a week
2. Quadriceps Stretch	2–3 stretches, 6 times a week	3 stretches, 6 times a week	3 stretches, 6 times a week
3. Upper Calf Stretch	2–3 stretches, 6 times a week	3 stretches, 6 times a week	3 stretches, 6 times a week
4. Lower Calf Stretch	2–3 stretches, 6 times a week	3 stretches, 6 times a week	3 stretches, 6 times a week
5. Middle and Lower Back Stretch	2–3 stretches, 6 times a week	3 stretches, 6 times a week	3 stretches, 6 times a week
6. Basic Crunches	2–3 sets, 6 times a week	3 sets, 6 times a week	3 sets; do either this exercise or Incline Sit-Up 6 times a week, alternating between the two
7. Twisting Trunk Curl Crunches	2–3 sets, 6 times a week	3 sets, 6 times a week	3 sets, 6 times a week

8. Upper Abdomen Crunches	2–3 sets, 6 times a week	3 sets, 6 times a week	3 sets, 6 times a week
9. Arm and Leg Raise	2–3 sets, 6 times a week	3 sets, 6 times a week	3 sets, 6 times a week
10. Shrug Roll	2–3 sets, 6 times a week	3 sets, 6 times a week	3 sets, 6 times a week
11. Heel Raises	2–3 sets, 6 times a week	3 sets, 6 times a week	3 sets, 6 times a week
12. Reverse Trunk Curl			3 sets, 6 times a week
13. Extended Arm Crunch			3 sets, 6 times a week
14. Vertical Leg Crunch			3 sets, 6 times a week
15. Incline Sit-Up			3 sets; do either this exercise or Basic Crunches 6 times a week, alternating between the two

STRENGTH-TRAINING EXERCISES (PP. 123–141)

EXERCISES	BEGINNER WEEKLY GOAL	INTERMEDIATE WEEKLY GOAL	ADVANCED WEEKLY GOAL
1. Squats	2–3 sets, 3 times a week	3 sets, every other day	3 sets, every other day
2. Lunges	2–3 sets, 3 times a week	3 sets, every other day	3 sets, every other day
3. Chest Press	2–3 sets, 3 times a week	3 sets, every other day	3 sets, every other day
4. Shoulder Press	2–3 sets, 3 times a week	3 sets, every other day	3 sets, every other day
5. Butterfly	2–3 sets, 3 times a week	3 sets, every other day	3 sets, every other day
6. Dumbbell Fly	2–3 sets, 3 times a week	3 sets, every other day	3 sets, every other day
7. Biceps Curl	2–3 sets, 3 times a week	3 sets, every other day	3 sets, every other day
8. Triceps Extension	2–3 sets, 3 times a week	3 sets, every other day	3 sets, every other day
9. One-Arm Row	2–3 sets, 3 times a week	3 sets, every other day	3 sets, every other day
10. Lateral Raise	2–3 sets, 3 times a week	3 sets, every other day	3 sets, every other day
11. Leg Press		3 sets, every other day	3 sets, every other day
12. Leg Extension		3 sets, every other day	3 sets, every other day
13. Leg Curl		3 sets, every other day	3 sets, every other day

14. Upright Row	3 sets, every other day	3 sets, every other day
15. Incline Press	3 sets, every other day	3 sets, every other day
16. Thumbs Down		3 sets, every other day
17. Frontal Raise	3 sets, every other day	3 sets, every other day
18. External Rotation		3 sets, every other day
19. Lat Pull-Down	3 sets, every other day	3 sets, every other day

AEROBIC EXERCISE (PP. 114–117)

AEROBIC WORKOUT	BEGINNER WEEKLY GOAL	INTERMEDIATE WEEKLY GOAL	ADVANCED WEEKLY GOAL
Regular Workout (your choice) at a 7–8 intensity	31 minutes or as much as you can do, 5 days a week	46 minutes, 5 days a week	61 minutes, 5 days a week
Double Workout (your choice) at a 6–7 intensity	62 minutes or as much as you can do, 1 day a week	92 minutes, 1 day a week	122 minutes, 1 day a week

WEEK 10
FUNCTIONAL EXERCISES (PP. 88–102)

EXERCISES	BEGINNER WEEKLY GOAL	INTERMEDIATE WEEKLY GOAL	ADVANCED WEEKLY GOAL
1. Hamstring Stretch	2–3 stretches, 6 times a week	3 stretches, 6 times a week	3 stretches, 6 times a week
2. Quadriceps Stretch	2–3 stretches, 6 times a week	3 stretches, 6 times a week	3 stretches, 6 times a week
3. Upper Calf Stretch	2–3 stretches, 6 times a week	3 stretches, 6 times a week	3 stretches, 6 times a week
4. Lower Calf Stretch	2–3 stretches, 6 times a week	3 stretches, 6 times a week	3 stretches, 6 times a week
5. Middle and Lower Back Stretch	2–3 stretches, 6 times a week	3 stretches, 6 times a week	3 stretches, 6 times a week
6. Basic Crunches	2–3 sets, 6 times a week	3 sets, 6 times a week	3 sets, do either this exercise or Incline Sit-Up 6 times a week, alternating between the two
7. Twisting Trunk Curl Crunches	2–3 sets, 6 times a week	3 sets, 6 times a week	3 sets, 6 times a week

8. Upper Abdomen Crunches	2–3 sets, 6 times a week	3 sets, 6 times a week	3 sets, 6 times a week
9. Arm and Leg Raise	2–3 sets, 6 times a week	3 sets, 6 times a week	3 sets, 6 times a week
10. Shrug Roll	2–3 sets, 6 times a week	3 sets, 6 times a week	3 sets, 6 times a week
11. Heel Raises	2–3 sets, 6 times a week	3 sets, 6 times a week	3 sets, 6 times a week
12. Reverse Trunk Curl			3 sets, 6 times a week
13. Extended Arm Crunch			3 sets, 6 times a week
14. Vertical Leg Crunch			3 sets, 6 times a week
15. Incline Sit-Up			3 sets; do either this exercise or Basic Crunches 6 times a week, alternating between the two

STRENGTH-TRAINING EXERCISES (PP. 123–141)

EXERCISES	BEGINNER WEEKLY GOAL	INTERMEDIATE WEEKLY GOAL	ADVANCED WEEKLY GOAL
1. Squats	2–3 sets, 3 times a week	3 sets, every other day	3 sets, every other day
2. Lunges	2–3 sets, 3 times a week	3 sets, every other day	3 sets, every other day
3. Chest Press	2–3 sets, 3 times a week	3 sets, every other day	3 sets, every other day
4. Shoulder Press	2–3 sets, 3 times a week	3 sets, every other day	3 sets, every other day
5. Butterfly	2–3 sets, 3 times a week	3 sets, every other day	3 sets, every other day
6. Dumbbell Fly	2–3 sets, 3 times a week	3 sets, every other day	3 sets, every other day
7. Biceps Curl	2–3 sets, 3 times a week	3 sets, every other day	3 sets, every other day
8. Triceps Extension	2–3 sets, 3 times a week	3 sets, every other day	3 sets, every other day
9. One-Arm Row	2–3 sets, 3 times a week	3 sets, every other day	3 sets, every other day
10. Lateral Raise	2–3 sets, 3 times a week	3 sets, every other day	3 sets, every other day
11. Leg Press		3 sets, every other day	3 sets, every other day
12. Leg Extension		3 sets, every other day	3 sets, every other day
13. Leg Curl		3 sets, every other day	3 sets, every other day

Exercise		
14. Upright Row	3 sets, every other day	3 sets, every other day
15. Incline Press	3 sets, every other day	3 sets, every other day
16. Thumbs Down		3 sets, every other day
17. Frontal Raise		3 sets, every other day
18. External Rotation		3 sets, every other day
19. Lat Pull-Down	3 sets, every other day	3 sets, every other day

AEROBIC EXERCISE (PP. 114–117)

AEROBIC WORKOUT	BEGINNER WEEKLY GOAL	INTERMEDIATE WEEKLY GOAL	ADVANCED WEEKLY GOAL
Regular Workout (your choice) at a 7–8 intensity	33 minutes or as much as you can do, 5 days a week	48 minutes, 5 days a week	63 minutes, 5 days a week
Double Workout (your choice) at a 6–7 intensity	66 minutes or as much as you can do, 1 day a week	96 minutes, 1 day a week	126 minutes, 1 day a week

WEEK 11
FUNCTIONAL EXERCISES (PP. 88–102)

EXERCISES	BEGINNER WEEKLY GOAL	INTERMEDIATE WEEKLY GOAL	ADVANCED WEEKLY GOAL
1. Hamstring Stretch	2–3 stretches, 6 times a week	3 stretches, 6 times a week	3 stretches, 6 times a week
2. Quadriceps Stretch	2–3 stretches, 6 times a week	3 stretches, 6 times a week	3 stretches, 6 times a week
3. Upper Calf Stretch	2–3 stretches, 6 times a week	3 stretches, 6 times a week	3 stretches, 6 times a week
4. Lower Calf Stretch	2–3 stretches, 6 times a week	3 stretches, 6 times a week	3 stretches, 6 times a week
5. Middle and Lower Back Stretch	2–3 stretches, 6 times a week	3 stretches, 6 times a week	3 stretches, 6 times a week
6. Basic Crunches	2–3 sets, 6 times a week	3 sets, 6 times a week	3 sets; do either this exercise or Incline Sit-Up 6 times a week, alternating between the two
7. Twisting Trunk Curl Crunches	2–3 sets, 6 times a week	3 sets, 6 times a week	3 sets, 6 times a week

8. Upper Abdomen Crunches	2–3 sets, 6 times a week	3 sets, 6 times a week	3 sets, 6 times a week
9. Arm and Leg Raise	2–3 sets, 6 times a week	3 sets, 6 times a week	3 sets, 6 times a week
10. Shrug Roll	2–3 sets, 6 times a week	3 sets, 6 times a week	3 sets, 6 times a week
11. Heel Raises	2–3 sets, 6 times a week	3 sets, 6 times a week	3 sets, 6 times a week
12. Reverse Trunk Curl			3 sets, 6 times a week
13. Extended Arm Crunch			3 sets, 6 times a week
14. Vertical Leg Crunch			3 sets, 6 times a week
15. Incline Sit-Up			3 sets; do either this exercise or Basic Crunches 6 times a week, alternating between the two

STRENGTH-TRAINING EXERCISES (PP. 123–141)

EXERCISES	BEGINNER WEEKLY GOAL	INTERMEDIATE WEEKLY GOAL	ADVANCED WEEKLY GOAL
1. Squats	2–3 sets, 3 times a week	3 sets, every other day	3 sets, every other day
2. Lunges	2–3 sets, 3 times a week	3 sets, every other day	3 sets, every other day
3. Chest Press	2–3 sets, 3 times a week	3 sets, every other day	3 sets, every other day
4. Shoulder Press	2–3 sets, 3 times a week	3 sets, every other day	3 sets, every other day
5. Butterfly	2–3 sets, 3 times a week	3 sets, every other day	3 sets, every other day
6. Dumbbell Fly	2–3 sets, 3 times a week	3 sets, every other day	3 sets, every other day
7. Biceps Curl	2–3 sets, 3 times a week	3 sets, every other day	3 sets, every other day
8. Triceps Extension	2–3 sets, 3 times a week	3 sets, every other day	3 sets, every other day
9. One-Arm Row	2–3 sets, 3 times a week	3 sets, every other day	3 sets, every other day
10. Lateral Raise	2–3 sets, 3 times a week	3 sets, every other day	3 sets, every other day
11. Leg Press		3 sets, every other day	3 sets, every other day
12. Leg Extension		3 sets, every other day	3 sets, every other day
13. Leg Curl		3 sets, every other day	3 sets, every other day

14. Upright Row	3 sets, every other day
15. Incline Press	3 sets, every other day
16. Thumbs Down	3 sets, every other day
17. Frontal Raise	3 sets, every other day
18. External Rotation	3 sets, every other day
19. Lat Pull-Down	3 sets, every other day

AEROBIC EXERCISE (PP. 114–117)

AEROBIC WORKOUT	BEGINNER WEEKLY GOAL	INTERMEDIATE WEEKLY GOAL	ADVANCED WEEKLY GOAL
Regular Workout (your choice) at a 7–8 intensity	35 minutes or as much as you can do, 5 days a week	50 minutes, 5 days a week	65 minutes, 5 days a week
Double Workout (your choice) at a 6–7 intensity	70 minutes or as much as you can do, 1 day a week	100 minutes, 1 day a week	130 minutes, 1 day a week

WEEK 12
FUNCTIONAL EXERCISES (PP. 88–102)

EXERCISES	BEGINNER WEEKLY GOAL	INTERMEDIATE WEEKLY GOAL	ADVANCED WEEKLY GOAL
1. Hamstring Stretch	2–3 stretches, 6 times a week	3 stretches, 6 times a week	3 stretches, 6 times a week
2. Quadriceps Stretch	2–3 stretches, 6 times a week	3 stretches, 6 times a week	3 stretches, 6 times a week
3. Upper Calf Stretch	2–3 stretches, 6 times a week	3 stretches, 6 times a week	3 stretches, 6 times a week
4. Lower Calf Stretch	2–3 stretches, 6 times a week	3 stretches, 6 times a week	3 stretches, 6 times a week
5. Middle and Lower Back Stretch	2–3 stretches, 6 times a week	3 stretches, 6 times a week	3 stretches, 6 times a week
6. Basic Crunches	2–3 sets, 6 times a week	3 sets, 6 times a week	3 sets; do either this exercise or Incline Sit-Up 6 times a week, alternating between the two
7. Twisting Trunk Curl Crunches	2–3 sets, 6 times a week	3 sets, 6 times a week	3 sets, 6 times a week

Exercise			
8. Upper Abdomen Crunches	2–3 sets, 6 times a week	3 sets, 6 times a week	3 sets, 6 times a week
9. Arm and Leg Raise	2–3 sets, 6 times a week	3 sets, 6 times a week	3 sets, 6 times a week
10. Shrug Roll	2–3 sets, 6 times a week	3 sets, 6 times a week	3 sets, 6 times a week
11. Heel Raises	2–3 sets, 6 times a week	3 sets, 6 times a week	3 sets, 6 times a week
12. Reverse Trunk Curl			3 sets, 6 times a week
13. Extended Arm Crunch			3 sets, 6 times a week
14. Vertical Leg Crunch			3 sets, 6 times a week
15. Incline Sit-Up			3 sets; do either this exercise or Basic Crunches 6 times a week, alternating between the two

STRENGTH-TRAINING EXERCISES (PP. 123–141)

EXERCISES	BEGINNER	INTERMEDIATE WEEKLY GOAL	ADVANCED WEEKLY GOAL
1. Squats	2–3 sets, 3 times a week	3 sets, every other day	3 sets, every other day
2. Lunges	2–3 sets, 3 times a week	3 sets, every other day	3 sets, every other day
3. Chest Press	2–3 sets, 3 times a week	3 sets, every other day	3 sets, every other day
4. Shoulder Press	2–3 sets, 3 times a week	3 sets, every other day	3 sets, every other day
5. Butterfly	2–3 sets, 3 times a week	3 sets, every other day	3 sets, every other day
6. Dumbbell Fly	2–3 sets, 3 times a week	3 sets, every other day	3 sets, every other day
7. Biceps Curl	2–3 sets, 3 times a week	3 sets, every other day	3 sets, every other day
8. Triceps Extension	2–3 sets, 3 times a week	3 sets, every other day	3 sets, every other day
9. One-Arm Row	2–3 sets, 3 times a week	3 sets, every other day	3 sets, every other day
10. Lateral Raise	2–3 sets, 3 times a week	3 sets, every other day	3 sets, every other day
11. Leg Press		3 sets, every other day	3 sets, every other day
12. Leg Extension		3 sets, every other day	3 sets, every other day
13. Leg Curl		3 sets, every other day	3 sets, every other day

14. Upright Row	3 sets, every other day
15. Incline Press	3 sets, every other day
16. Thumbs Down	3 sets, every other day
17. Frontal Raise	3 sets, every other day
18. External Rotation	3 sets, every other day
19. Lat Pull-Down	3 sets, every other day

AEROBIC EXERCISE (PP. 114–117)

AEROBIC WORKOUT	BEGINNER WEEKLY GOAL	INTERMEDIATE WEEKLY GOAL	ADVANCED WEEKLY GOAL
Regular Workout (your choice) at a 7–8 intensity	37 minutes or as much as you can do, 5 days a week	52 minutes, 5 days a week	67 minutes, 5 days a week
Double Workout (your choice) at a 6–7 intensity	74 minutes or as much as you can do, 1 day a week	104 minutes, 1 day a week	130 minutes, 1 day a week

5

MAKING THE TRANSITION TO REAL LIFE

WHEN YOU HAVE COMPLETED the 12-Week Total Body Makeover program, the first thing you should do is congratulate yourself. Congratulate yourself for staying committed, for being honest with yourself and taking responsibility for your behavior, for exhibiting a great deal of willpower, and, not least, for exhibiting a great deal of physical strength. The Total Body Makeover program is not a walk in the park, so if you have seen it through to the end, you are to be celebrated!

What now? I hope that the time you have spent exercising and following the five simple rules for better eating has made you want to continue to do what it takes to stay in great shape. That doesn't mean that you need to keep working out as vigorously as you have been the last 12 weeks. You might remember that at the outset of the program I encouraged you to think like an athlete. Athletes typically stay in good shape year round, but they don't necessarily maintain their peak condition all twelve months. They go through intense training periods, then back off a bit to give their bodies a break.

Here's what I suggest you consider when contemplating where to go from here. First, look at how much time you are willing and able to devote to exercise. How will working out fit into your life? Be realistic about your time parameters and reassess your goals. Then consider your options. If you're up for it, you can continue exercising at the same pace where you left off at the program's end. This might be a particularly good idea when it comes to certain aspects of strength training. Once you build up to a point where you can lift a particular amount of weight and do a certain number of sets and repetitions, why let it go? If you can do 3 sets of 10 repetitions of biceps curls using, say, 15-pound dumbbells, there's no reason to start doing less.

If you were able to do considerably more than the basic eight strength-training exercises, you may want to consider reducing the number of exercises you do as well as the number of times per week you work out, depending on your progress and your own goals. If you advanced to performing strength training every other day, dropping back to three days a week will be fine. If you went beyond performing the first eleven functional exercises, you can eliminate some of the exercises and do them only three times a week. Then again, you may just want to stay where you are—and I especially recommend that you continue to strength train at the same or nearly the same effort.

I also hope that if you decide to scale back your aerobic exercise, you won't cut the duration of your workouts by more than 10 to 15 percent. Staying fairly close to where you left off in week twelve, and maintaining the same pace, will allow you to preserve all the hard-earned cardiovascular strength and endurance that you gained during the program. If, to solve a time crunch, you need to reduce the number of days per week you work out, still try to perform aerobic exercise at least four and preferably five days a week. The best-case scenario: keep the frequency and intensity of your workouts the same, and cut the duration slightly if you have to.

When it comes to how you transition your eating, you have a few options. If you haven't yet met your weight loss goal, assess how you're doing. If your weight is still creeping down, even if less than a pound a week, consider just continuing to exercise and sticking with the Five Simple Eating Rules outlined in chapter 3. This may be all you need to eventually reach your goal.

When and if you consider choosing a formal eating plan, it should be either because you have hit a plateau where you're not losing anymore or you simply feel that your eating is still out of control and that you need structure. Diets definitely have their place; they can help you organize your eating by limiting the amount and/or type of food you eat so that you aren't susceptible to making bad choices. Diets can even recondition your taste buds by requiring that you eat foods you normally wouldn't. If you lack discipline, diets can help rein in your free-spirited approach to eating. Some diets, because they cause you to lose a fairly ample amount of weight in the beginning (although this weight isn't necessarily body fat), can even give a program that's stalled a nice jump start.

Later in this chapter, I'll give you some information aimed at helping you find a diet that suits your lifestyle. But before I get to that, I want to encourage you, whether you end up going on a diet or not, to continue following the Five Simple Eating Rules. While these rules were mostly intended to help you lose an optimal amount of body fat during the 12 weeks, they were also meant to help you develop long-term healthy eating habits. In other words, this is how you should be eating for life. And the rules, after all, are simple—so stick with them! Stop eating two to three hours before your bedtime. Have a nutritious breakfast every morning. Drink at least eight glasses of water a day. There is some leeway on the no-alcohol rule; I don't expect you to abstain from drinking forever. But remember that alcohol adds calories, can impair your judgment about what you eat (not to mention many other things), and, the day after make your exercise routine feel more difficult.

Remember, always continue to make eating a conscious act. Eating for reasons other than physical hunger may be something that you will continue to deal with, but this is a fight worth winning. Stopping emotional eating is key to retaining the control over your life that you have gained during the last 12 weeks. So stay vigilant. Use your journal and periodically go back to the strategies for getting a grip on emotional eating on page 158. Always *think* before you eat; asking yourself whether you're really hungry or not and reflecting on why you feel the need to eat can really make a difference.

Surveying the Diets

All diets work. By that I mean that any diet you go on can help you lose weight as long as it reduces your calorie intake. Although the people who create different diets would like you to believe that their diet, and their diet alone, really does the job, *all* diets can help you slim down.

The question is, for how long?

That's really the crux of the matter. To see dramatic results, you need to *stay* on a diet. To see dramatic, long-term results, you need to, first, stay on the diet; then second, be able to transition into a way of eating that is healthier and lower in calories than the way you ate before. Any diet will work in the short term, but a good diet will work for a lifetime. It will be satisfying enough to keep you on it long enough to reach your goal weight, and, most important, it will help you discover a better approach to eating. By my definition, if a diet is a good one (and it doesn't even have to be a "diet" in the strict sense of the word, it can also just be a style of eating) it will change your mind about what you "have to have" and what you can live without. A good diet makes you think differently about food and transforms the way you eat beyond just a few weeks. Even if you don't end up following the diet's maintenance plan (if it offers one) once you've hit your goal, the weeks you spent following the diet should help change your mind-set about food so that you don't return to your old way of eating. A good diet, when it's over, will leave you a healthier eater.

So which are the good diets? Beyond a few standard requirements—that the diet be safe, for instance—a diet's merit depends on how it suits your own particular lifestyle, tastes, and goals. The diet that helps your sister or best friend get great results won't necessarily be the one that will help you do the same. Even if your goal isn't to lose weight at all but just to learn to eat more healthfully, the diet that's going to help you is the one that matches your sensibility: it should appeal to your food preferences and individual nutritional needs and not make demands on you that—even if you are highly motivated and committed to losing weight—you don't think you can keep. If your schedule makes it impossible to consume six small meals a day, a diet that depends on eating often probably won't help you lose weight. No diet is easy and they all require compromise, but you can better set yourself up for success if you choose one that's as closely suited to your tastes and lifestyle as possible.

Something else that's critical to consider when choosing a diet is how that diet will fuel you for exercise. The amount of carbohydrate you need to take in each day is dictated by how active you are—carbs are the muscles' preferred fuel—and that in turn should dictate the type of diet you go on. If you're very, very active, you are going to need an eating plan that provides an ample amount of carbohydrates. But no matter how much you work out, especially now, when low-carbohydrate diets are all the rage, make sure that the carb consumption allowed by a diet will match your activity level.

The fact that there are so many weight loss and nutrition plans available says something about the very nature of dieting. One way to look at it is that bookstore shelves sag with diet books because there is no such thing as a miracle weight loss cure. If a single diet provided the secret to a healthier America, we could all pack our bags and go home, confident that the obesity epidemic would decline as rapidly as it has arisen. But that's far from what's happening. You could say that the failure of each of those diets to help overweight Americans is probably due to one of two factors: either the person following the diet has not completely committed to making healthy changes in her life, or she has selected a diet that simply doesn't suit her.

We are all different. We don't all dress alike, like the same books, frequent the same restaurants. Why, then, should we all expect to be able to eat the same way? A high-protein menu that a friend finds suits her tastes to a T may actually be unpalatable to you. It happens all the time, yet many people expect that what works for one person will automatically work for another. Believe me, it's not a moral failing if your cousin lost on Atkins but you can't follow it for more than two days. What's more, we all have different body types and energy needs. If you're working out consistently, a diet that works for someone who manages to get in 20 minutes only sporadically—or does no exercise at all—isn't likely to bring you success.

The stories you have been reading throughout this book reinforce the point that a diet needs to suit the individual. Almost everybody had a different road to success, including the approach to eating that helped them make their bodies over. Likewise, when O, The Oprah Magazine asked readers to respond to the contract I designed for the January 2003 issue, the multitudes of women who wrote in to tell us their stories described varying dietary approaches to weight loss. Some women were using my books as a guide; some had figured out their nutritional needs on their own. Some used the Atkins plan; others relied on Curves or the South Beach Diet to point the way.

Since I work with clients who follow a wide range of different eating plans, I wasn't surprised to learn that many different diets work. One of the most interesting examples of this is a recent study conducted at Tufts University. The study involved 160 men and women who were asked to follow one of four diets: the high-protein, high-fat Atkins diet; the very-low-fat, high-carbohydrate Ornish diet; or the more moderate Weight Watchers or Zone diets. Those who stuck it out for a year (half the Atkins and Ornish volunteers dropped out, as did about 35 percent of the Weight Watchers and Zone dieters) lost about 10 to 12 pounds. They all also reduced their risk factors for heart disease, such as their cholesterol and insulin levels. The researchers concluded that all the diets did the job—as long as the dieters stuck with them.

Stick-to-itiveness, of course, was the bottom line. Nobody loses weight by throwing in the towel. But how, you might be wondering, can diets that are so fundamentally opposite—the Ornish diet, for instance, allows only about 10 percent fat, while the Atkins plan places no limit on it—all help people to slim down? There's a simple answer: calories. All the diets in the study help you reduce your calorie intake, and when it comes to weight loss, that's what really counts. No matter what type of food you eat, you will lose weight only if you burn more calories than you consume. So if a diet gets you to cut back, it is more than likely going to work.

I think the best diets are those that aren't drastic but rather provide a reasonable plan for long-term healthy eating. While it's not an ideal approach, in my opinion, you can also follow a diet that is meant to give quick, short-term results as long as you're aware that when the diet ends you're going to need to exercise and eat in moderation to maintain the results. Transitioning is essential if you hope to keep the pounds from piling back on. Also keep in mind that a diet that causes you to lose a lot of weight right away (generally water weight) might not be the kind of diet you'd want to stay on for long. For instance, it's not a good idea to stay on a diet that allows you to eat only a miniscule amount of carbohydrates or one that restricts your fat intake to a few grams a day for longer than a few weeks, though one of these types of diets may help you jump-start a lifelong program of more calorie-conscious eating and work your way into healthier habits.

Changing the way you eat is one of the most difficult challenges there is, so it's especially important to select a diet you can live with. One of the ways people tend to choose diets is that they hear about a friend or relative's success or read about how the diet helped some celebrity get into enviable shape. What I want you to do instead is read about ten of the most popular diets here, then make your choice based on what is most likely to lead to *your own* success. I've studied them to find out their pros and cons and who they're likely right for. That, I hope, will help you cut to the chase and figure out which plan will work best for you. As you read, ask yourself which diet sounds as if it's doable for you. Which have drawbacks that may bother you, which don't? Which has advantages that will make it fit more easily into your lifestyle?

You might also want to look beyond the eating plans that I mention here; you don't have to be limited to these. If none of them seems right, explore some of the other available options. I will caution you, however, to look for a diet that won't compromise your health while you lose weight. A diet shouldn't, for instance, be so restrictive that it limits your intake of the nutrients you need. Everyone's calorie requirements are different, but if you're living on not much more than a baked potato and salad each day, it's not a healthful diet for anyone (at least not for more than a day or two). Likewise, a healthful diet won't require you to take handfuls of supplements each day or spend your time making complicated liquid concoctions. A healthful diet won't have you depending on only one or two foods either. Look for a plan that offers you a variety of different foods and doesn't require that you spend a lot of money or purchase hard-to-find foods. You want something that you can see living on, in one form or another, for a lifetime.

Step-by-Step Diets Aren't for Everyone

Some people really like the idea of having all their meals and snacks mapped out for them: for them, taking the decision making out of eating also takes some of the temptation out of eating. But you don't have to follow a "diet" to lose weight or change your eating habits for the better. If you know the basics about what constitutes healthy eating—which I'm guessing that you may, you can create your own plan. That's what many of the successful people whose stories are chronicled in these pages did, including Renee. Here's her story.

Devising Her Own Diet
Renee's Story

Over the last seven years, I have transformed myself. I had been obese for my entire life despite the fact that the rest of my family was thin and I grew up in a genuinely happy and loving home. I suppose I just overate and made the wrong food choices, although in retrospect my mom fed me healthy, balanced meals and I really couldn't pinpoint any differences in the way I ate from any other kids my age. It seemed that I was just meant to be fat.

But as any obese person knows, no matter how much you seem to be taking things in stride, hidden underneath the fat was a depressed, unhopeful person suffering from the way she was treated. Growing up, I faced daily ridicule from friends, teachers, strangers, and anyone else who didn't seem to notice that, despite being obese, I had feelings and a heart of gold.

Finally, when I was in college, I decided it was time to make a change. After the holiday break, I went back to school and just decided to start eating healthfully and to exercise. I started with a very-low-fat diet, cutting out fast foods and going to the gym with friends. I took the exercise part very slowly. At first I could ride the bike at the gym for just 10 minutes. It was horrible and embarrassing, but I kept at it and little by little I was able to increase my strength and endurance. I would challenge myself to stay with it by saying to myself, "Just keep going for one more song," and inevitably I would prove to myself that I could do it.

During this phase, I didn't follow any particular diet plan per se; I just gathered information from magazines and other resources. I'd even go up to people in the gym who I thought seemed very fit and ask them questions like "What do you eat for lunch?" It took me two years to lose 150 pounds, though when I look back it seemed like it happened fast. The hardest part was having my mental self catch up to my physical self. Like most women, I am very tied up in my body image, and sometimes I'd find that I'd forget how far I'd come and beat myself up over a slipup even though I did get a lot of positive feedback. They even put my picture up on a display board at the gym!

Still, I wasn't done yet. I still felt that I wanted to lose more weight, and in January 2003 I renewed my commitment by signing the contract offered by Oprah and Bob in O magazine. It was at this time that my mother also suggested that I see a doctor who practiced alternative medicine. Up until that time I had been eating tons of low-fat and nonfat carbohydrates and lots of processed foods. The doctor said I was probably insulin-resistant from overloading my body with so many carbohydrates, and because I'd sworn off dietary fat, my body was likely holding on to every bit of body fat that it could.

I went home from his office and overhauled my eating habits. I started by cutting down on carbs, except for salad greens and the small amount of carbohydrates in cheese. I began eating lean proteins, healthy fats, and no processed food. I upped my water intake and supplemented my diet with vitamins and minerals. By the next day I already felt less bloated, and after two weeks I had dropped eight pounds. What's more, for the first time in my life, every single stomach problem I had miraculously disappeared. I was so full of energy (I still am!), and as the weeks went on I began to see some muscle development from all the hard work I'd been doing at the gym.

Ultimately, although I lost only about 10 pounds in this second phase, my body reshaped itself. I feel like a million bucks, and I also feel like I don't have to be a fat-free freak anymore. For the first time in seven years I can enjoy the foods I love so long as I stay away from most carbs and processed foods with sugar and additives. My husband got to take me out for a breakfast of healthy omelettes for the very first time. I used to go to restaurants and just sit while everyone else ate because there were no fat-free selections on the menu. No more!

My new, healthier approach to eating has also given me the energy I need to train for the many fitness events I enter. Along with exercising about six days a week—1 hour and 10 minutes of cardio, 40 minutes of weights—I run a lot of races and do charity "climbs" in buildings in Chicago. I have run a half marathon as well as climbed to the top of the Hancock Building and the Sears Tower (103 flights in 24 minutes!). I feel like I'm catching up with what I missed out on in high school.

Both phases of my journey have been life-altering, and now, after my renewed commitment to a healthy lifestyle, I can say that my spiritual and emotional being are whole. I am happier, radiant, and at peace. My husband and I seem to be having more fun, and my enthusiasm for life has been renewed.

When I embarked on this wild ride, I made a solid decision: "I'm going to do it, and I'm not going to stop." But I have also had to remind myself that there would be bad days and frustration along the way. I still have days when I feel fat, but I know it's going to pass. And it always does!

DIET REVIEW

The Atkins Diet by Robert C. Atkins, M.D.
(www.atkins.com)

The Premise

This is perhaps the most famous low-carbohydrate, high-fat and protein diet around. It's known primarily for allowing dieters to indulge in foods, such as butter and steak, that have traditionally been crossed off the dietary roster. Robert Atkins died in 2003, but he left reams of information about why he (and many others) believe that the Atkins plan works. Here are the main theories behind the diet:

- A low-carbohydrate approach to eating keeps blood sugar stable and thus reduces hunger pangs and cravings.
- When you eat a traditional, carbohydrate-rich diet, the body stores the carbohydrates in the liver and muscles in a form called glycogen. It then draws on that glycogen for energy. When your carbohydrate intake is severely restricted, your body quickly depletes your glycogen stores and is forced to burn more body fat for fuel. In short, if you eat fewer carbohydrates, you'll burn more stored body fat.
- A diet high in carbohydrates, says Atkins, promotes insulin resistance, which in turn promotes the storage of body fat. A low-carbohydrate diet, on the other hand, lowers insulin levels, not only reducing fat storage but also reducing the risk of diabetes.
- By promoting fat burning, the Atkins diet creates a process called lipolysis, the by-products of which are substances known as ketones. Some experts warn that overproduction of ketones can be harmful, but Atkins says that there is no evidence of this and that lipolysis breaks the cycle of excess insulin production and its result, fat storage. Ketones also help suppress the appetite.
- When it's burning fat (as opposed to carbohydrates), the body burns more calories overall. That increase, together with the fact that the diet helps decrease your appetite so you eat less, means you'll burn more calories than you take in, resulting in weight loss.
- Some studies have shown that the less carbohydrate consumed, the more

weight lost—even when there is no reduction in calorie intake. In other words, you can eat the same amount of total calories, but if you're proportion your diet, cutting out most carbohydrates, you will still shed pounds.

The Eating Plan

The diet is divided up into four parts. The first phase lasts a minimum of 14 days and includes three regular or four to five small meals a day. It allows for liberal consumption of meat, eggs, fish, and poultry, as well as pure fats, such as healthy vegetable oils, and fats traditionally considered not so healthy, such as mayonnaise and butter. (At least that was the original idea. Lately the Atkins camp has been discouraging unlimited consumption of saturated and hydrogenated fats.) Only 20 grams of carbohydrate are allowed a day, which translates into 3 cups of salad or vegetables. On the forbidden list: fruit, bread, cereal, pasta, grains, starchy vegetables, dairy products (other than cheese and butter), nuts, seeds, and beans. Caffeine is not allowed either, but vitamin and mineral supplements are.

Phase II, for ongoing weight loss, bumps up the amount of carbohydrates you can eat (per day) by 5 grams each week for a total of 25. You can also add some fruit—berries only—to the mix. Depending on how you're doing, seeds, nuts, wine, legumes, and a few other items not allowed in Phase I can also be added. The next phase, premaintenance, allows you to add 10 grams of carbs a day each week until you find that you are no longer losing. The number of carbs that you stop at is where you stay in the final phase, lifetime eating. That number is typically anywhere from 40 to 60 grams.

How Exercise Fits In

Atkins emphasizes the importance of exercise and also contends that the diet will give you more energy and thus help you exercise more. I haven't seen this to be the case, so I'd say that the jury is still out on that one. The truth is, if you work out fairly hard, you'll probably find that the lack of carbohydrates on this diet leaves you without sufficient energy.

The Advantages

Research has shown that most people who lose weight on the Atkins plan experience improved cholesterol and triglyceride levels. And most people do lose weight on Atkins; in fact, they tend to lose more weight than people who go on low-fat diets (although they also gain it back more quickly). From a motivation standpoint, that may be a plus. (However, much of the weight lost is water weight, and ultimately that's not what you want.) Another advantage of the diet is that many people who go on it say that they're not as hungry as usual. That makes sense: the diet's mainstays, fat and protein, take a long time for the body to digest, so it's likely that this diet actually does keep hunger at bay. Also, ketones do reduce appetite, as Atkins claims.) The diet is not intended to be a low-calorie diet, but in most cases it does get dieters to cut enough calories to cause a substantial number of pounds to budge. (You aren't, after all, allowed to eat sweets, crackers, pasta, rice, or soft drinks, so if those were the mainstay of your diet, you're going to pare down your calorie intake.) In that sense, the Atkins plan can be a fairly painless way to lose weight—as long as you can keep it up for the time you need to, then transition into a solid exercise and moderate eating program.

The Drawbacks

Despite the improvements in cholesterol and triglyceride levels, the generous amount of saturated fats allowed on this diet is still worrisome. Will those fats have a long-term impact that we don't know about (studies usually follow dieters for only six months to a year)? Recently spokespeople for the company have said that the diet has been misunderstood: although it does allow for a large proportion of fat (up to 60 percent of total calories), only a third of that is supposed to be saturated fat. Perhaps their message will get across, but in the meantime, most people are interpreting the diet as a steak-and-egg extravaganza, and that could mean trouble. Many health experts are united behind the idea that, for heart health, we need to keep our intake of saturated fats (and hydrogenated fats called trans fats) to an absolute minimum. Atkins counters with the fact that studies have shown that people who followed the plan lowered their cholesterol and triglyceride levels; however, there is no saying whether or not these health improvements will hold up long term. A few people who went on the diet have had heart problems, though it is uncertain whether the diet is to blame. Nobody really knows if it's healthy to stay on the diet for an extended period of time. (The diet has also been linked to an increased risk of developing kidney stones.)

Another potentially problematic aspect of the diet is the lack of fruits and vegetables. Although produce is severely limited only in the beginning phases of Atkins, I still find it troubling that the diet doesn't emphasize produce when science tells us that diets high in fruits and vegetables are instrumental in disease prevention. In addition, although eating starches (and particularly refined starches) can certainly be overdone, diets high in whole grains have been shown to help prevent disease—and to be linked to a healthier body weight. The Atkins diet makes up for the lack of fiber by recommending a supplement or bran or flax. That doesn't sound like the best way to get fiber, but if you're going to follow the diet, it's probably a good idea to adopt this strategy.

Something else it's important to consider about this diet is that its very restrictive approach to carbs can make it difficult to fuel your body properly if you're consistently working out vigorously. Last, many people complain that when they start increasing their carbohydrate intake, they gain back weight almost instantaneously.

Who This Diet Is Right For

If you're someone who likes meat, fish, and poultry and finds fats hard to give up, Atkins may well work for you. Likewise, if carbohydrates are your weakness, the plan may help you slow down and get a grip on those cravings. I'd advise against following the diet if you have a personal or family history of heart disease. At the very least, if heart trouble is an issue, make sure you talk to your physician before going on the diet. Also note that a diet that has you dependent on a lot of meat, poultry, and seafood will generally mean there'll be more kitchen work involved—and more cost, too.

The South Beach Diet by Arthur Agatston, M.D. (www.southbeachdiet.com)

The Premise

Like many other diet gurus, Dr. Agatston, a Miami-based cardiologist, bases his plan on the idea that refined carbohydrates are at the root of today's obesity epidemic. What makes the South Beach Diet somewhat different is that Agatston does not ban all carbohydrates; he even acknowledges that many of them are good for you. His diet is based not on "low-carb" eating or "low-fat" eating but rather on the notion that you should eat only "good" carbs and "good" fats. This isn't to say that pasta and bread lovers can rejoice; you are still expected to keep carbohydrate eating to a minimum, and the first phase is very restrictive in terms of carbs. Likewise, you are not given free rein to eat all the eggs (considered a good fat) and olive oil you want. The diet, though, does include these foods, and one of Agatston's aims is to keep you from feeling deprived and to ensure that you don't feel hungry.

The main bit of science that drives the South Beach Diet is the glycemic index. A food's glycemic index (GI) is the amount that it raises blood sugar compared with how much the same quantity of white bread would raise it (which is to say a lot). Foods with a high GI cause a spike in blood sugar and an equally quick decline, which, Agatston says, leads to more hunger and subsequent weight gain. Since highly processed carbohydrates almost always have a high GI, those are the foods that are largely banished from this diet.

You are not, however, encouraged to load up on foods such as cheese and red meat in their place (though you can eat them in moderation). One way in which this diet differs from Atkins is that it's designed to keep your intake of unhealthy saturated fats low. Agatston also does not think it's a good idea to limit carbs so severely, as long as the carbohydrates you eat are fiber-rich.

The Eating Plan
The first two weeks of this diet are designed to help you stabilize your blood sugar. It allows you to have three moderate-size meals, plus two snacks and dessert at night. In this phase, you eliminate bread, rice, potatoes, pasta, baked goods, anything containing sugar, fruit, and all alcohol from your diet. (The doctor promises that your cravings for these foods will disappear.) What you can have during this phase is normal-size helpings of meat, poultry, and seafood, eggs, cheese, nuts, and lots of vegetables, including salads with olive oil dressings. In the second phase, you can reintroduce some of the banned foods, such as pasta, whole grain bread and cereal, potatoes, and fruit. The final phase, which you go into when you've achieved your goal weight, is basically your choice, but with the hope that you will continue eating healthy fats and a small amount of high-fiber carbs that are low on the glycemic index.

How Exercise Fits In

Dr. Agatston encourages exercise and also offers a few diet modifications for those who are doing long-duration workouts. But exercise isn't really a big factor in this plan, and the doctor notes that you don't have to exercise to succeed on the South Beach Diet.

The Advantages

This diet has a (deserved) reputation as being healthier than the Atkins diet because it's stricter about the types of fat that dieters are allowed and concentrates on wholesome, nutritious foods. While the first phase is pretty restrictive, the diet allows you to build healthy habits so that if you follow the general premise of the diet—substantially reducing your intake of processed carbohydrates—you will have a pretty good dietary road map for life.

The Drawbacks

There has been some criticism of Dr. Agatston's reliance on the glycemic index because the index doesn't always take into account the way in which foods are eaten. Carrots, for instance, have a high GI—but only in large amounts. If you eat one carrot, it won't raise your blood sugar the way its GI number indicates. Likewise, some high-GI foods are eaten along with other foods (a cracker and a dollop of peanut butter, for instance) that slow their ability to cause a rise in blood sugar. But all that science won't matter so much if you don't like the diet, which has been a problem for some people who found that, contrary to promises, they still had carb cravings. This diet also involves a lot of cooking, which may be a drawback for some people (although the recipes are pretty nice). Another downside, again probably only for a minority of people, is that the recipes sometimes call for products such as liquid egg substitute, processed vegetable oil spreads, and sugar substitute, which some find unappealing.

Who This Diet Is Right For

If you know you eat too many processed carbs—crackers, cookies, white bread, pasta, white rice—this diet provides a good opportunity to learn how to live without them. And you can do so without having to live on meat and chicken, which may be a relief if you find it hard to swallow all that protein.

It's still low-carb living, but it's less drastic than other low-carb diets. This diet is also a good pick for people who like to cook, especially since many of the recipes are from some of Miami's top chefs. Be advised that this is not the cheapest diet you could select. The recipes often call for high-end ingredients (such as crab, fresh herbs, Asian condiments) and this can be costly.

Dean Ornish's Lifestyle Program by Dean Ornish, M.D. (www.ornish.com)

The Premise

Despite the onslaught of low-carb diets, Ornish, a cardiologist, has steadfastly stuck with his argument that very-low-fat eating is the best path to both weight loss and heart health. While he agrees that Americans should significantly reduce their intake of refined carbohydrates (such as white bread and white rice), he believes it's important to get abundant quantities of whole grains as well as fruits and vegetables. He also bases his plan on the notion that to lose weight you need to eat fewer calories than you burn and that the easiest way to reduce your calorie intake is to consume less fat (fat has 9 calories a gram, protein and carbohydrates both have 4). Perhaps the best way to describe Ornish's program is holistic. For good health and weight loss, the plan also emphasizes exercise, stress management, and connecting with other people.

The Eating Plan

This diet is largely vegetarian, based on fruits, vegetables, whole grains, beans, and soy products. It does, however, include eggs, and you have the option of adding lean meats if you like. But there are almost virtually no added fats (taking an omega-3 fatty acid supplement is advised) in the recommended recipes. Salad dressings are made without oil. Quesadillas are made with nonfat cheese. Even brioche, a classic recipe for an egg-rich bread, is made with the whites of the eggs only. The plan offers sample menus as a guide-line—you do not have to count calories or worry about portion sizes.

How Exercise Fits In

Ornish considers exercise a critical part of the plan and recommends walk-ing 30 minutes, three times a week, at a pace of 50 to 80 percent of your maximum heart rate. The eating plan will likely provide you with enough carbs to keep you fueled for exercise.

The Advantages

The very-low-fat nature of this diet makes it pretty certain that you will end up reducing your calorie intake quite a bit. You'll probably still stay well within a healthy level of calories but also cut enough to make the pounds come off. Another plus is that there is some sound research to show that the diet helps reverse some of the problems, such as high cholesterol, that are associated with heart disease.

Because there is no calorie counting or measuring, Ornish's plan is easy to follow. And while you'll probably do best if you make the recipes provided, you can probably stick to the diet if you just always opt to leave the fat out of foods you make from your own recipes (or buy fat-free foods). Another plus is that the menus are packed with fresh fruits and vegetables. You'll probably get more than five servings of produce a day on this diet. That, combined with the fact that there are very few processed foods on the menus, may make you feel as if you are truly eating from nature's bounty.

The Drawbacks

There is very little protein on this plan, which may make some people feel deprived. This is especially true if you don't like tofu or other soy products, because, while you have the option of lean meats, it helps if you like soy. The very-low-fat nature of this diet may also leave you feeling hungry. Ornish counters that the many high-fiber foods on the diet are filling, but for some people there's no substitute for fat.

Who This Diet Is Right For

Because of the diet's proven ability to counter heart disease, this is a good choice for people who are actually suffering from the condition or who are at risk. Fruit and vegetable lovers may also appreciate this diet. If you really like fresh foods and aren't so attached to fat that you will miss it desperately, you will probably do well on this program. Those who like to cook may also enjoy this diet because the recipes are sophisticated in flavor, though not terribly hard to make, and you may learn some culinary tricks for reducing fat.

Ornish's diet is also a good choice for people who like food guidelines but don't want to have to follow a diet to the half tablespoon. You will probably also like this program if you are seeking other ways (i.e., stress management and connecting to other people) to improve the quality of your life.

The Zone Diet by Barry Sears, Ph.D. (www.drsears.com)

The Premise
The Zone is another diet that is based on the idea that eating too many carbohydrates is both unhealthy and a major cause of excess poundage. Sears, who is a biotechnologist, defines "the Zone" as a metabolic state in which the body works at peak efficiency. If you're in the Zone, he says, you will experience painless fat loss, optimal wellness, and increased energy. Much of Sears's program hinges on controlling the body's balance of eicosanoids, hormones that he says impact the body's ability to deflect disease. To keep the balance of good and bad eicosanoids favorable, Sears claims that's it necessary to make sure that every meal and snack you eat has a makeup of 40 percent carbohydrates, 30 percent protein, and 30 percent fat. That's higher in protein and lower in carbs than in many diets, but still relatively moderate in fat.

The Eating Plan
You won't find a typical meal plan in the Zone, but rather guidelines to help you adhere to the 40–30–30 balance of carbohydrate, protein, and fat. To begin with, you calculate your protein requirements by determining your body fat percentage using a mathematical worksheet, a scale, and a tape measure. Once you know your body fat percentage, you factor in how active you are to come up with your daily allotment of protein grams. From there you figure out your carbohydrate and fat gram requirements. Within these parameters, you can then take your pick of foods, with some stipulations. The Zone restricts "bad" saturated and hydrogenated fats, such as butter and vegetable shortening, and recommends that you go very easy on unfavorable carbohydrates—those that register high on the glycemic index, such as bread, pasta, grains and potatoes and produce such as papaya, corn, and carrots. A few more rules of the road map: Eat five times a day, try not to consume more than 500 calories per meal or 100 calories per

snack, and always try to maintain the 40–30–30 ratio. Sears also recommends adding an omega-3 fish oil supplement to the diet.

How Exercise Fits In

Interestingly, Sears has tested the Zone on athletes, most notably the Stanford swim team, which took eight gold medals at the 1992 Olympics. He claims that the diet is on the cutting edge of sports nutrition, though others aren't so sure. There have been some reports of active people who felt the diet didn't provide them with enough energy due to its lack of carbohydrates, the muscles' main source of fuel. Sears devotes a chapter of the book to exercise and incorporates activity when determining the amount of protein each individual Zone follower requires.

The Advantages

The Zone is a low-calorie diet and therefore will probably help you lose weight. It wisely limits unhealthy fats and basically calls for lots of healthy foods such as fruits, vegetables, and lean forms of protein. While the 40-30-30 parameters are rigid, the list of foods you are required to eat is not. Unlike other diets, the Zone is not wildly restrictive in some areas and wildly libertine in others. That may make it more achievable for a lot of people.

The Drawbacks

Sears's eicosanoid hypothesis has never been proven and has been questioned by other experts. That said, there's nothing harmful about the eating philosophy that has come out of his theories. What may prove to be more of a problem is that this diet requires that you do a lot of measuring and package reading in order to determine how many grams of carbohydrate, fat, and protein you are eating (though Sears also offers a less exact way of eyeballing food to determine the proper nutrient ratio). It may also be difficult to meet the 40-30-30 food ratios at every meal (let alone snacks). Last, a diet of 40 percent carbohydrates is still pretty low if you exercise vigorously consistently.

Who This Diet Is Right For

If you like to be on your own without having to follow a set menu, the Zone may be for you. It tends to be pretty low in calories, so you'll have to see if you can feel satisfied on the plan; otherwise you may just end up cheating, then beating yourself up for failing, when the reality is that you just weren't following the right diet for your needs. If you dislike having to pay close attention to the details of what you're eating, you should probably pass on this one.

Eating for Life by Bill Phillips (www.eatingforlife.com)

The Premise
The Eating for Life "recipe" for eating right has four components: the right foods, the right amounts, the right combinations of foods, and the right times. It's not a diet per se, but rather a guide to eating nutritiously—as the title indicates, "for life." Phillips doesn't believe in calorie counting or in carb counting—he is anti-low-carb dieting—and thinks that eating a balanced diet is far more effective. A lot of his ideas are based on common sense, and various studies that show that eating often and eating the right combinations of foods increases the burnoff rate of the foods consumed.

The Eating Plan
The first part of Phillips' plan, the right foods, involves a fairly long list of authorized foods in all categories (protein, fats, and carbs). These foods should make up the mainstay of your diet, and you can eat them however you like, though in reasonable portions. That's where the second part of the recipe, the right amounts, comes in. Phillips provides a way to eyeball portions so that you don't have to measure them. The third component, the right combos, encourages you to include a portion of protein and carbohydrate in each of your meals. The last component, the right times, refers to eating six meals a day. (The extra meals are generally protein shakes or bars.) Eating for Life advocates sticking to this program six days a week, then having a free day when you can eat anything you like. Phillips also encourages you to plan your meals the day before so that you know what you're going to eat and not make the mistake of just grabbing whatever's available.

How Exercise Fits In
Eating for Life is an adjunct to Body-for-Life, a comprehensive fitness program, so Phillips is obviously a big proponent of exercise. A lot of the eating plan is

developed from his own experience, and since he is an avid exerciser himself, it takes into consideration the needs of people who work out vigorously.

The Advantages

There is nothing kooky about Eating for Life, and its guidelines are simple and easy to follow. They don't require wrapping your mind around any esoteric information, and they allow you a lot of freedom in what you choose to eat. The recipes provided with the plan are nice and not hard to make.

The Drawbacks

There aren't a lot of specifics for those who need a little more direct guidance. Phillips also advocates eating a biggish dinner, which could get people who tend to take things to extremes into trouble, as could the free day. Noncooks beware: you don't have to cook to stay on this plan, but it's a good idea since all the meal plans are based on Eating for Life recipes. Likewise, you don't have to buy the nutrition shakes recommended by the program, but you're strongly encouraged to do so.

Who This Diet Is Right For

If you are very disciplined and prefer to have some flexibility in a diet plan, Eating for Life is a good choice. It's a good program for exercisers and for people who like to cook. It may, however, be onerous for those who don't have the time to work in six meals a day.

WeightWatchers
(www.weightwatchers.com)

The Premise

Weight Watchers combines an eating plan with group meetings. Although you don't have to attend meetings to use the plan, support and camaraderie are one the hallmarks of Weight Watchers, and some people find them to be the key to their success. The diet is based on the idea that you should be able to choose the foods you like to eat and that you will lose weight if you eat those foods according to a points plan: each food corresponds to a points value, and you can consume a certain number of points each day. Along with points guidelines, dieters are provided with reams of information designed to educate them about healthy eating.

The Eating Plan

The number of points you are allotted depends on how much you weigh, but each person gets an amount that will most likely lead him or her to lose one to two pounds a week. Everybody also gets 35 flex points for the week, which can be used to cover slipups or just a desire to eat a little more. Though you can choose whatever foods you want as long as you stay within your points parameters, Weight Watchers helps you determine the right mix of nutrients and portion sizes and encourages you to select foods according to its "8 Healthy Habits" guidelines.

How Exercise Fits In

Weight Watchers encourages people to exercise and offers plenty of fitness tips but leaves it up to you to weave exercise successfully into your life. To inspire dieters, it awards points for activity that can be swapped for food. It doesn't offer enough exercise help, in my opinion, but because it does offer so much else, I think the Weight Watchers eating program teams up nicely with my exercise program.

The Advantages

One of the biggest advantages of Weight Watchers is the meetings, where you can find like-minded people struggling with the same issues you are as well as inspirational people who have been successful. The diet allows for a lot of flexibility, yet offers boundaries so that you don't have to figure out your daily food allotment yourself. Some research also suggests that a fairly high percentage of people who go on the program lose weight and keep it off.

The Drawbacks

There are really very few drawbacks to this program. One might be the required weighing of food and point calculations. In addition, some may find that it doesn't offer dramatic enough results, but that's just the point: it's based on the premise that slow and steady wins the race.

Who This Diet Is Right For

People who like an interactive program or who need support will find this to be a great choice. It will also probably help if you are willing to do some work yourself, such as reading the information the program provides and making choices based on it. You could easily fill up all your points with ice cream, for instance, but you'll be less likely to do so if you stay on top of all of Weight Watchers' recommendations. This diet may also appeal to vegetarians—it's one of the few plans that provides vegetarian alternatives. And again, I think the Weight Watchers program pairs up nicely with my exercise program. Together they provide a very comprehensive plan.

The Ultimate Weight Solution Food Guide by Dr. Phil McGraw (www.drphil.com)

The Premise

Dr. Phil's food guide is meant to go hand in hand with his *The Ultimate Weight Solution: The 7 Keys to Weight Loss Freedom*. Weight loss, he believes, begins with psychological change, then segues into a change in eating habits. Dieters first need to change their taste preferences, then build their diet around what he calls high-response-cost, high-yield foods. These foods are nutrient-dense, encourage slow eating, are satisfying, and prevent cravings and hunger pangs. The opposite—low-response-cost, low-yield foods—need to be avoided because they usually cause uncontrolled eating.

The Eating Plan

The plan begins with a 14-day Rapid Start Plan that includes three meals and two snacks a day. The plan is designed to help you learn to lose your taste for high-fat, high-sugar foods or at least feel satisfied by healthier choices. The plan has about 1,100 to 1,200 calories; 30 percent from protein, 45 percent from carbohydrates, and 25 percent from fat. Next, dieters move on to the High-Response-Cost, High-Yield Weight Loss Plan, which is almost exactly the same as the Rapid Start Plan. The final portion, Maintenance, allows for slightly more food than either plan. In general, the menu plans are full of lean protein sources, whole grains, healthy fats, unlimited vegetables (except for starchy ones, of which you can eat a little bit), and a few servings of fruit. The menu plans don't include desserts.

How Exercise Fits In
Although he devotes little time to it, Dr. Phil strongly advises using exercise to help with weight loss (and good health). He doesn't gear his menus toward exercisers, but active people should find that they provide adequate fuel.

The Advantages
The foods recommended on this plan are not exotic, but neither are they boring, and how you want to prepare them is left up to you. The nutrient breakdown of the menus is moderate and healthy and unlikely to leave anyone feeling fatigued. If you don't like the menus, *the Ultimate Weight Solution Food Guide* gives you guidelines for creating your own.

The Drawbacks
The concept of high-response-cost, high-yield foods can be a little confusing. These are essentially foods that are healthy, yet the idea is kind of complicated by the jargon. If you just see them as foods allowed on the diet (and their counterparts, low-response-cost, low-yield foods, as not allowed), you may fare better. There are no recipes provided, so you're on your own as to how to prepare the allowable foods.

Who This Diet Is Right For
This is another program that is moderate and easy to follow and can be turned into a plan you can follow after you reach your goal. It will probably appeal to you if you don't want to be too hemmed in by menu plans (the ones here are flexible) and you aren't looking for something that will give you a dramatic start to weight loss.

Curves by Gary Heavin and Carol Colman (www.curvesinternational.com)

The Premise
The Curves diet is an adjunct to a fitness plan offered at the women-only Curves fitness centers, a chain with outposts around the world. Because

Heavin believes that the same diet doesn't work for everybody, Curves actually offers dieters a choice between two different eating plans. One is for women (the diet, like the club, is aimed at women) whom Heavin and Colman call "carbohydrate sensitive"; the other is for women who are "calorie sensitive." The carb-sensitive plan is high-protein, low-carbohydrate. The calorie-sensitive plan is more liberal in the amount of carbohydrates you can eat but, more restrictive caloriewise. One of the main ideas behind both plans is that many people, either because of their natural body type or because of persistent on-again, off-again low-calorie dieting, have a very slow metabolism. The diets are designed to increase your metabolism so that once you've lost the weight you want, you can go back to your normal way of eating. The diet's tagline is "Permanent results without permanent dieting."

The Eating Plan
If you are following the carbohydrate-sensitive plan, you can eat unlimited amounts of lean meats, cheese, eggs, seafood, and poultry and no more than 20 grams of carbohydrates a day in the form of six meals a day. The diet also includes unlimited "free" foods (mostly vegetables) and one protein shake per day. Depending on how much you have to lose, you stay in phase one for a week to two weeks, then move to phase two, which allows for more food and is five weeks long. Although you're told you can eat unlimited amounts of protein, the diet actually provides serving sizes and you will probably do better if you stick to them (though blank menu forms are available to allow you to devise your own menu).

If you are following the calorie-sensitive plan, you can eat 1,200 calories a day and no more than 60 grams of carbohydrates. You're also advised to get 40 percent of your calories from protein. The plan includes six small meals a day, and you are also allowed the same free foods and daily protein shake as the carb-sensitive people. In phase two you increase your calorie intake to 1,600.

Once you've reached your goal weight on either diet, you can move into phase three and eat 2,500 to 3,500 calories. First, though, it's recommended that you do a "metabolic tune-up." This involves eating normally and, when you gain back three pounds or so, going back to phase one for 72 hours. You do this a few times, and after a few months you will be able to maintain your weight by having to go back to phase one for only a few days once in a while. In other words, you can pretty much eat as you want and then use the diet to rein your weight back in when necessary.

All dieters are encouraged to take quite a hefty amount of vitamin and mineral supplements.

How Exercise Fits In

Exercise is an imperative adjunct to this program. Heavin believes that you can achieve permanent weight loss only if you increase your muscle mass through strength training. The Curves exercise program involves a particular type of strength training called circuit training, which involves moving from one weight station to another (eight in all) with 40 seconds of aerobic recovery in between. The authors recommend 30 minutes of exercise a day, three days a week. Many women have found that this exercise program really works for them, although I think that for long-term maintenance, exercising three days a week should be the bare minimum and that more intensive strength-training and aerobic workouts will make you fitter.

The Advantages

It's true that not all people who are overweight have the same response to food, so it's helpful, I think, that Curves offers two different diet plans. Heavin also provides a questionnaire to help you figure out whether you are carbohydrate- or calorie-sensitive. The low-carb plan is solid and doesn't encourage dieters to eat all kinds of unhealthy foods the way some others do. And both menus are fairly easy to follow: the recipes are simple, and you should be able to find all the foods without any problem. The diets anticipate plateaus, and Curves offers advice on how to overcome them.

The Drawbacks

I am skeptical about the idea that you can return to your previous way of eating and still maintain your weight loss. Also, the calorie counts called for both on and off the diet might not be right for everybody. Twelve hundred calories a day (the amount in the calorie-sensitive diet) may be too low for some people who are larger and who are exercising vigorously. On the other hand, other people may find that the maintenance level of 2,500 to 3,500 calories a day is too high. While I'm sure that the idea is to get people to continue to eat healthfully when they go off the diet, Heavin makes it seem as if you can just go back to eating as you did before, which for most people isn't a good idea. Finally, the idea of a metabolic tune-up, where you eat as much as you want, gain weight, then go back on phase one for a few days, doesn't seem like the healthiest approach to weight loss and maintenance.

Who This Diet Is Right For

The carbohydrate-sensitive program is a good choice for people who *don't* mind missing out on foods such as bread and crackers. The calorie-sensitive program is good for people who *do* mind missing out on foods such as bread and crackers. It's also good for people who can comfortably live on 1,200 calories a day, which is not all that many. To succeed on one of these diets, you should not be opposed to measuring your portions, which is required, or eating six times a day, another requirement. If you prefer a diet that's easy to follow—you do have to shop, but you don't have to scour specialty markets for ingredients—one of these diets will also work for you. The only downside of the simplicity is that the meals aren't terribly exciting, but if plain suits you—perhaps you even need plain food to retrain your palate—these fit the bill.

The Carbohydrate Addict's Diet by Dr. Rachael F. Heller and Dr. Richard F. Heller (www.carbohydrateaddicts.com)

The Premise

The Hellers believe that millions of people are overweight because they have a physiological imbalance called carbohydrate addiction. Their theory is that carbohydrate addicts' bodies release far more insulin than is necessary within a few minutes of their eating carbohydrates. This excess insulin interferes with the absorption of glucose and subsequently the body's hunger signals. The brain fails to detect the signs that the body is satisfied, so it creates a sensation of hunger. Some carbohydrate addicts feel hungry again (usually for sweets and other starchy foods) in two hours, as if they've never eaten at all. Some symptoms of carbohydrate addiction, the Hellers say, are a frequent focus on eating, lack of satisfaction, and feelings of fatigue, as well as anxiety, anger, and heightened emotionality.

Unlike other anti-carb diet proponents, the Hellers believe it's not just how many carbohydrate grams are eaten but how frequently carbs are eaten that matters. Eating lots of mini-meals and snacks, they contend, sets off the insulin response, inducing the body to store more fat and creating more hunger—if, that is, you are a carbohydrate addict. The authors concede that not everyone is and that their diet might not be right for all people who need to lose weight.

The Eating Plan

In general, the plan involves no weighing and measuring, allows for favorite foods (even things such as doughnuts and ice cream if you want) and while sample meal plans are offered, you are free to develop your own using the Carbohydrate Addict's Diet guidelines.

The diet begins with an entry plan that allows for two "complementary meals" and one "reward meal" a day. Complementary meals must be made up of food low in carbohydrates (no fruit allowed) and consist of average (3- to 4-ounce) servings of meat, fish, or poultry or two ounces of cheese and two cups of vegetables or salad. The reward meal is a "mini-feast"—a meal (but not a binge) that includes foods you enjoy, which can include anything, even alcohol and dessert.

After you complete the entry plan for one week, you weigh yourself and the amount you weigh determines the next plan you will follow (there are four of them). The diet plans aren't very different from the entry plan, adding in a snack here and a salad there. A few stipulations: no snacking at all (other than on the plan that allows one), and meals must be eaten within an hour.

How Exercise Fits In

In the small box that they devote to exercise, the Hellers say that activity is not an integral part of their weight loss plan. While they encourage dieters to exercise for good health and to feel good, they say not to do so to advance their weight loss goals.

The Advantages

You don't really have to do any measuring on this diet, and you can devise your own plan, which means the foods may be more to your liking. Though some recipes are included, you don't have to go out of your way to find special foods in order to follow the diet. The Hellers' approach, whether it is as scientifically grounded as they say or not (some say not), seems to help certain people fight cravings and reduce their hunger.

The Drawbacks

If you are not a carbohydrate addict, as described by the Hellers, this diet may not work for you. The reward meal may be a good idea for some people, but others may be tripped up by its liberal nature and overeat. And I worry that the no-snack rule may make some dieters flag: if you're low on energy, you're not going to have the get-up-and-go you need for exercise. One other thing that strikes me about the rationale behind the diet is that many of the symptoms the Hellers attribute to carbohydrate addiction sound to me like emotional eating. I think it's important that if you're going to follow this diet, you not ignore the fact that you may need to deal with the emotional and not just the physical reasons you eat.

Who This Diet Is Right For

This is a good diet for people who don't need structure and prefer to devise their own menus. It's also a good diet for people who don't feel the need to snack and can maintain their energy on just three meals a day. If you have a lot of weight to lose and really need a strict plan, I'd discourage you from following this diet. If, however, you just need a little help in cleaning up your diet and can benefit from focusing on making two meals a day superhealthy, the Carbohydrate Addict's Diet may be an acceptable choice.

Sugar Busters! by H. Leighton Steward, Sam S. Andrews, M.D., Morrison C. Bethea, M.D., and Luis A. Balart, M.D. (www.sugarbusters.com)

The Premise

This diet is based on the idea that the overeating of sugary, highly processed food is the main culprit behind weight gain. Like the creator of the South Beach Diet, the authors propose eating low on the glycemic index scale to prevent insulin overload and subsequent fat storage. Yet while they believe that dieters should not eat certain carbohydrates (and especially sugar) at all, they think that other diets go too low and that it's important to eat healthy carbohydrates because of the nutrients they add to the diet.

Another theory behind the development of this diet is that meals abundantly rich in carbohydrates suppress glucagons, substances released from the pancreas that helps the body burn stored fat. A high-protein meal, on the other hand, causes an increase in glucagon secretion.

The Eating Plan

It might actually be more appropriate to call this a lifestyle plan than a diet because the authors simply provide some suggestions (in the form of lists of acceptable foods for meals and snacks) rather than any step-by-step menu plans. Essentially, though, dieters are advised to eat high-fiber vegetables and whole grains, meats that are lean and trimmed, and reduced-fat dairy products. Unlike some other carb-conscious plans, this one allows you to have fruit (though not all types of fruit). Without being specific, the diet recommends moderate portion sizes, finishing your evening meal by 8 P.M., and eating at least three meals a day. In contrast to the Carbohydrate Addict's Diet, which contends that eating too often causes insulin to get out of control, Sugar Busters! maintains that long intervals between meals alter the body's response to insulin and promote fat storage.

How Exercise Fits In

Like many other authors of diet books, the Sugar Busters! group says that you don't need exercise to lose weight on their program. Nonetheless, they recommend at least 20 minutes a day 4 days a week. They also mention that if you are a marathon runner or "exercise fanatic," the diet might not be right for you since you may need to eat more carbohydrates than the diet allows for.

The Advantages

This is a very reasonable program without any drastic measures. You will probably feel very satisfied if you follow the authors' lists of acceptable foods, and while there aren't many dessert options, you can at least have something. I like that the authors encourage a reduction in refined carbohydrate eating—most people do eat too many refined carbs—but don't severely restrict your carbohydrate intake.

The Drawbacks

You really have to process the information provided by the authors; you can't just flip to the back and follow the menu plans right away (there are none). That may be a good thing—you will learn along the way—however, it can be a drawback if you need more guidance. This plan doesn't really change at all, which again could be a good thing (it teaches you how to live with healthy eating, not to go onto and off of a diet) or a bad thing (there's no jump start with tangible results for those who need a little motivation), depending on how you look at it. The authors don't provide any numbers, so it's a little difficult to know how much you're supposed to eat.

Who This Diet Is Right For

If you would like to reduce your carbohydrate intake but can't bear the thought of eating next to no carbs, this diet offers a happy compromise. Self-motivators will also like this diet because you really have to depend on yourself to figure out a food plan. Nobody holds your hand, and there's no measuring or carb or calorie counting. Likewise, anyone who really wants to learn some nutrition basics and not just follow steps may find this diet helpful. The diet includes many recipes from gourmet restaurants around the country and even around the world (there's one from Saudi Arabia), so if you like to experiment in the kitchen, this may be for you.

Getting the Life You Want—and Deserve

This 12-week program is, on the surface, about changing your body and improving your health. But it's also about so much more. After devoting twenty-two years of my life to working with people trying to transform themselves, I have found that the process is always less about the amount you exercise and what you eat than about looking at your life and having the courage to change it.

In a sense, the Circle of Life, described on page 155, really tells it all. The circle lets you ask yourself, "What's important to me?" and "How can I make each area of my life better?" Improving your eating and exercise habits is just a slice of it. The real challenge is to bring all the parts of your life into balance. When you do that, a fit, healthy body just naturally follows.

The successful people you've read about throughout this book have all discovered this. They're masters of addressing all different aspects of their lives and finding ways to improve them. And interestingly, most of them had no idea that this would be the result when they started out on their journeys. Most of them were just trying to change the way they looked. Yet all of them ending up changing their lives in significant and often dramatic ways.

So with them as inspiration, let me leave you with these thoughts: Work toward fulfilling your life on all levels. Care deeply for yourself, and have the wherewithal to do what it takes to make yourself happy. Go out and claim the life you deserve! If you can do this, you'll be sure to succeed.

INDEX